Cognitive Behavioral Therapy

The Complete Guide to Using CBT to Battle Anxiety, Depression and Regaining Control over Anger, Panic,and Worry.
By: Daniel Patterson

Table of Contents

Therapy Techniques on Your Own

Make Sure That You know:

Conclusion

Introduction

You might have heard of cognitive behavioral therapy (CBT)—the evidence-based psychotherapy procedure dedicated to changing unwanted ideas and behaviors—before. It seems to be cited in virtually every informative article on the web: Insomnia issues? Try CBT. Struggling with trauma? CBT will provide help. For stress, depression, very low self-esteem, anxiety about traveling, etc., CBT may be your answer. There's a high probability that you have received CBT or that you may even know somebody that has.

So what is CBT? Does it genuinely alleviate emotional distress and how does it achieve this? Yes, it does and the exact methods may be puzzling for some.

What exactly is CBT?

CBT is just one of the dozens of remedy options utilized in psychotherapy. It truly is centered upon the premise that a lot of life's issues come from defective notions (that is precisely where "cognitive" stems from) and behaviors. By deliberately altering them to healthier, more successful objectives, we could ease distress. In training, CBT is commonly composed of pinpointing both the controversial views and behaviors, and replacing them with responses that are wholesome.

CBT is a type of communicating therapy that helps to identify difficult thoughts, and also supports many people to mostly know how to pattern their thinking and even their behaviors, ultimately improving their way of feeling. This investigates the relationship that occurs between behaviors, feelings, and thoughts. Therefore, it arises from two very different schools of psychology: Cognitive therapy, and behaviorism. The roots of these can be trailed to two models.

CBT is also defined as the joining together of both behavioral and cognitive therapies, with empirical support strong enough to be deemed as medical care for many physiological disorders.

CBT also focuses on building a person's personal skills, or matching skills that will empower them to become conscious of feelings and thoughts, and identifying solutions. It also has a way of impacting people's perception, aiding the improvement of bad feelings by replacing behaviors and beliefs. CBT is different from other traditional methods of talk therapy as it gives a determined prominence to the individual's acquired skills and the use of assignments. This therapy aims not just to solve any individual's current problem or to work on the negativity of their thoughts but to assist in improving the toolkit of the individual to become efficient in solving problems that may arise in the near future.

How does CBT work?

CBT, unlike psychoanalytic and psychodynamic therapies, is a short-term approach that usually takes as little as 6 sessions, or even up to 20 sessions. All through every session, you and your therapist might identify situations and circumstances within your life that might have caused your low mood, or contributed to it. This is when your current way of thinking and your distorted perception can be tackled and identified. You might be encouraged to save journals to keep records of each of your life events and your reactions to them. This might also assist the therapist to break down and identify your thoughts and reactions, which may include:

- All for nothing thinking which views the world as black or white.

- Rejecting the positives, which might disqualify every positive experience and feeling that you've had.

• Overgeneralization, which means drawing broad conclusions regarding a particular event.

• Automatic negative thoughts i.e. when you experience scolding thoughts.

• Taking things just too personally i.e. thinking that some things happen due to what you say, what you've done, or a feeling that everyone's actions are mostly directed to you.

• Unrealistically reducing or increasing the usefulness of every event, which means building up or bringing things down in a way that might not match the real world.

• Focusing on a negative issues i.e. dwelling on things to the point whereby your general perception is very dark.

What Types of Problems can CBT Solve?

CBT can be employed for stress, depression, injury, self-esteem problems, ADHD, inferior communication, or unrealistic expectations of one's partner, to name a few. When it's a problem that entails notions and behaviors, CBT acts as a cure.

Why is CBT Popular and Trusted?

A reason for CBT being so popular and trusted is that it's been analyzed so broadly. It's worth researching about as it highlights fast and solution-oriented interventions; its intention is always to generate distinct and quantifiable adjustments in notions and behaviors, and it is seen as a goldmine for therapists.

What Occurs at a CBT Session?

At the start, the therapist is likely to mention a method of payment, the cancellation policies, the aims for the therapy, the client therapy report, plus a summary of the client's problems. From then on, the discussions will be around the battles that the client faces and how to alleviate them.

The therapist and client interact to generate an action program for whatever problem the client is facing. An activity plan signifies that they establish the debatable notions and behaviors, discover an easy method to improve them and produce a way to execute this plan.

What's CBT Training Like?

CBT relies on offering an instant and efficient decrease of outward symptoms. Regular training may incorporate exercises a keeping a diary of ideas and feelings. It may also incorporate methods aimed a particular subject, examining relevant publications or searching out circumstances to employ your new strategy.

How Long Does a CBT Remedy Usually Last?

One of the highlights of CBT is that it is centered on eradicating signs and indicators as speedily as possible, on average in a month or two—depending on the patient's ability to focus in therapy, and the quantity and seriousness of their problems. Brevity is crucial for the particular approach; an essential feature that stands CBT out from other therapies.

Are there any CBT Methods Which People can use aside from Actual Therapy Sessions?

Perhaps you have kept a gratitude diary? Have you thought about tracking your junk food intake? Have you ever monitored your sleep patterns and its quality?

If you've done any of these, you are already employing a few of the fundamentals of CBT into your daily activity. However, personalized and structured therapy remains the best.

A lot of information will be shared in this book to help anyone showing symptoms that CBT could alleviate. The importance of CBT cannot be overemphasized, and so let's delve deeper!

Chapter 1: The History of Cognitive Behavioral Therapy (CBT)

CBT has become well-known over the years as many people are now very much aware of its use and efficacy in treating known disorders like depression and anxiety. This is not a new therapy whatsoever, and it has a structure that makes it easy to measure the results—factors that have made it easy to have many successful clinical trials and as a treatment that is endorsed and used for the UK's NHS.

Spiraling Towards Success

In the 1960s, a psychiatrist by the name of Aaron T. Beck treated individuals who were suffering from depression. He wanted to understand better the legitimacy of psychoanalysis methods made famous by Sigmund Freud. Though Beck started doing some research and experiments with the hope of verifying the relevant treatments techniques, he discovered that the methods had very little or no positive effects on patients that were depressed. Upon finding this great stunning revelation, Beck had no other choice than to develop other new and effective methods to assist his patients. As a result, with the aid of other known, celebrated figures like Albert Ellis, Beck developed the treatment methods of CBT.

Since Dr. Beck first started treating his depressed patients with his newly developed therapeutic methods, CBT became one of the highest regarded treatments for mental health.

With the modernized structure of CBT today, there are other various therapeutic activities that psychiatrists can use not just to help their patients prevail over depression but also other health disorders, such as obesity, addiction, and anxiety.

While it might be easy to think that CBT can only be used by medical professionals in treating those with mental health struggles, this isn't the case. The structure of CBT is built on fundamental psychological beliefs that can be applied to anyone.

The Foundational Framework of CBT

Before looking in depth at the other ways that we can use CBT's tools and exercise for our personal development, it's important to gain a better understanding of the treatment's methods and their underlying structure.

For those that do not have prior knowledge of CBT, the most important thing is that CBT therapists work with patients at the cognition and behavioral levels—the "C" and "B" parts of CBT. Beyond this fundamental point, it's imperative to briefly examine the four concepts that stand as the background of which CBT is built upon—The CBT triangle, automatic thoughts, dysfunctional thinking, and the cognitive model.

The CBT triangular model explains how an individual's emotions, thoughts, and behaviors affect everyone. A CBT therapist always sees the triangle as one of the psychological facts that guides all of humanity.

The CBT therapist starts working with patients to form the treatment methods with the understanding that all individuals' behaviors, thoughts, and emotions affect one another continuously, at all times. For example, when an individual begins to think badly, there will be severe repercussions at the behavioral and emotional level. Likewise, if an individual behaves destructively, there will be severe ramifications at the emotional and cognitive level.

Since cognitive thoughts do not affect our behaviors and emotions, our emotions also affect behaviors and emotions; everyone can take actions that are life-affirming at both the behavioral and cognitive levels in ways that increase the feeling of subjective well-being.

The cognitive concept of the CBT model explains how specific circumstances and situations lead to a chain reaction of body sensations, thoughts, behaviors, and emotional responses. When an individual suffers from social anxiety, they are usually in a high-pressured environment; they will be anxious about cognitions that guide their behavior. The thoughts and emotions of social anxiety have a way of influencing one another; individuals will take steps to take themselves out of the situations. The model explains to us that these situations cause thoughts that allows emotions to alter our behavior.

Lastly, the CBT concept of automatic thoughts and dysfunctional thinking are areas where a mental ailment develops. While psychiatrists and psychologists of various schools of thought will not agree on everything, they all agree that there is a flow of seemingly automatic thoughts flowing from our brains. When working with people that have a mental illness, a CBT therapist will point the finger towards every negative cognition or dysfunctional patterns of thinking as the culprits causing a behavioral and emotional disturbance.

Behavioral Therapy Roots

Treatments for behavioral disorders have been available for a long time. In the early 1900s, Pavlov, Skinner, and Watson were all early supporters of behavioral treatments. Behaviorism is rooted in the idea that every behavior can be trained, measured, and also changed. It also connotes the fact that our environment has a way of shaping our behavior.

Behavioral therapy came about at first in the 1940s, as a response to WWII veterans needing support in adjusting back into "normal" life and dealing with their horrific experience of war. It was used as a short-term therapy of anxiety and depression that corresponded with the research into how people learn to react emotionally and behave in different life situations. This confronts psychoanalytic therapy which was famous during the time and is considered as CBT's first wave.

The old behavioral therapy approach is no longer as commonly used as it was many years ago. Right now, we have a more collaborative approach to the treatment of cognitive issues, and it has proved to be more reliable.

Cognitive Therapy Roots

In the 1900s, an Australian psychotherapist's (Alfred Adler) concept of fundamental mistakes and the role they play in unpleasant emotions made him among the earliest therapists to deal with psychotherapy cognition. The work he carried out inspired the American psychologist Albert Ellis to change Rational Emotive Behavioral Therapy (REBT) in the 1950s. This is now known to be the earliest form of cognitive psychotherapy, and its fundamental idea is that a person's emotional discomfort comes from either their thoughts about an event or the event that happened itself.

In 1950-1960, the aforementioned psychiatrist Aaron T. Beck learned that most of his clients had internal communications (voices in their heads) during their therapy sessions. He also found that some clients also seemed to talk to themselves but didn't share with him what these voices said. For example, a client saying, "The therapist is quiet today. I wonder if he is not happy with me." And by that, they are already anxious about the result.

Automatic Thoughts in Cognitive Therapy

Beck knew that the usefulness of the link between feelings and thoughts. He then coined the phrase "automatic thoughts" to tell us what exactly was going on in our minds. He also found out that though many people are not conscious of these thoughts, they can learn to report and identify them; he discovered that people who are angry always have bad thoughts, and by uncovering and challenging these thoughts, there can be long-lasting positive changes. In other words, CBT assists people to come out of this automatic thought process.

In the 1960s, a series of studies empirically showed how cognition influences emotions and behaviors; this is also known as cognitive revolution and is also referred as CBT's second wave. It strictly stresses the importance that conscious thoughts play in psychotherapy.

Combining the Approaches

Behavioral therapies are also relevant in treating disorders like neurosis, but have not yet been able to overcome depression. As cognitive therapies have become more popular and psychologists are seeing more and success with them, the joining together of different approaches can be used to successfully treat panic disorders. CBT remains as placing greater emphasis on the individual's experience, belief, and feelings at every given moment.

Chapter 2: Is CBT the Right Therapy for You?

Are you puzzled about the various types of therapy that are available? If so, you are not alone. CBT is one of the best known forms of therapy, but how can it help you and what does CBT entail exactly?

Whenever I meet a client for the very first time, I ask questions about what they know about CBT and, most times, the response I get is quite the same: "Very little." This is not exactly a problem, though, as part of my job is to tell them how it works and also to take them through the process. Nevertheless, I'm sure there are more people than one realizes whom are in dire need of help and don't realize how CBT can be exactly what they need.

CBT is still relatively new and is respected everywhere because its fundamentals are based on a simple proposition that our thinking affects our feelings. This begins by developing a better understanding of how we usually think of ourselves and those around us, which might lead to an emotional disturbance.

Here, we will discuss ways in which different CBT strategies can help you to start thinking and behaving in a healthy and emotional way.

So, how will you know if CBT is appropriate for you?

I'll assume that you are reading this chapter because you are not feeling too well, and that you are struggling with your life and no longer feel your "normal" self. This might be a feeling that you have been noticing for a very long time or it might've been triggered recently. You might be aware that you are suffering from some depression or anxiety or you might also have anger issues. You might also be in a very tough personal situation, self-confidence is low or you feel alone.

Emotional problems can be in various forms, and one of the vital keys is to know if CBT can help. It can be very difficult to pull yourself together or snap out of how you feel—no matter how much you bottle it up, talk about it, or try as much as possible to ignore it, those negative thoughts and feeling always appear and seem to get worse each day. The positive, if this is how you feel, is that no matter how bad you feel, you can also change—CBT helps by establishing an equilibrium, and making necessary adjustments to make sure that things go back to normal for you, and that you develop a more helpful and positive perspective.

So, if you are looking for a therapy that follows a strategic and logical process, one that assists in changing and also moving forward the things that are holding you back, then CBT is a good option to explore. Unlike other psychoanalytic therapies that help to focus on things of the past, CBT discourses what happens presently—it takes what has happened in past events to help know or take into account why you are going through current emotional trauma, basically focusing on solutions and methods to bring about a long-term change. The philosophy that is learned can be applied through so many life circumstances.

Hence, CBT is very useful in the modern day, encouraging you to always be responsible for the way you feel, empower you with the emotional consciousness, providing effective ways to cope with difficult life challenges. We are not born with our feelings and thoughts, but they often develop as we begin to grow older, which can be influenced by our teachers, friends, our daily experiences, and parents. This will assist us to understand that we have the power to change our thoughts. And if our thoughts enhance the way we feel, we need to understand the sort of thoughts that leads us to unhelpful emotions, so that we can make the necessary changes.

A very important question to consider is how often you are used to "black and white" thinking in your life? "I must succeed. If I don't, I'm a failure," "that person did not smile back at me, so I know they don't like me." This unyielding, all-or-nothing tendency creates more pressure and is an example of a thought distortion that is more likely to be targeted for change, and to create alternatives that are more balanced.

Quick Checklist

CBT can help if:

- you want to learn and take control of your emotions
- you love the idea of a logical, scientifically-proven therapy that will help you change how you feel presently and also in the future
- you believe that change is possible even if it seems impossible at the moment
- you are happy to practice strategies between sessions
- you feel blocked and stuck

Chapter 3: The Daily Lifestyle Guide to CBT

There is a theory that if you do something consistently for 21 days it becomes a habit. CBT will help you inculcate good habits into your daily lifestyle, and you will become a better you.

Here are some guidelines that could help you, daily, to achieve your goals.

Pleasant Activity Scheduling

Pleasant activity scheduling is not as effective as behavioral therapy techniques but is particularly useful for those who are suffering from depression.

Try this: Write down the next 21 days on a piece of paper starting from today (Thursday, Friday, Saturday, etc.). For each day, schedule a pleasant activity—things that you love doing. It could be as easy as reading a chapter from a novel. An alternative method is to plan an activity for a day that will give you an edge and a sense of competence, accomplishment, and mastery. Also, pick something small that you wouldn't usually do—target anything that won't take you less than 10 minutes to accomplish. An improved method is to plan three nice activities every day; make it one in the morning, one at noon and the other one in the evening. Having events that bring high levels of positive emotions daily in your life will make you think less and be less negative.

Situation Exposure Hierarchies

Situation exposure hierarchy is doing things that you normally abstain from doing. For instance, an individual who has an eating disorder might have a list of forbidden foods, with ice cream topping the list and full-fat yogurt at the bottom. Someone who has social anxiety might decide that asking someone out on a date causes the highest anxiety, but asking someone for directions causes the least.

The idea of the hierarchy is to make a list of 10 items that cause the most anxiety or negative trigger, with 10 being the most. For example, for the eating disorder above, the ice cream would be 10 and the yogurt 1. The logic is to work your way up the list from the smallest to the highest—to expose yourself to these things in order to face your fears.

Imagery Based Exposure

A version of imagery exposure involves having a recent memory that provokes intense negative emotions. For example, a student of clinical psychology that was given a critical report by the supervisor—in imagery based exposure, the person might bring the scenario while the report was given to mind and remember vividly (example, what the room looked like, the tone the supervisor used).

They will also attempt to precisely label thoughts and emotions that they have experienced during interactions and what their urges are (example, to get angry or run out of the room to cry). In extended imagery exposure, the person will have to keep visualizing images until the level of discomfort is being reduced to half of its a starting point (say from 8/10 to 4/10).

Imagery based exposure can assist counter ruminations just because it assists in making intrusive, painful experiences that can likely trigger rumination, due to this, it also leads to a decrease in avoidance coping. When a person is not comfortable by the intrusive experiences gained, they will be able to choose healthier coping actions.

CBT Method

Setting realistic goals and understanding how to solve problems (e.g., engaging in more social tasks; learning how to be deciphered).

In some instances, CBT is most effective when it's done along with different remedies, including antidepressants or other drugs.

Also, fairly little is understood regarding the process of fitting treatments (such as CBT) to individuals. Skilled practitioners, though, are often ready to accommodate CBT to a vast array of circumstances and people.

Example 1

Jenny has been fighting with problematic drinking for decades. She understood there could be alcoholic beverages at the upcoming company party. She also knew her co-workers sometimes put a lot of pressure on her to drink. Jenny along with also her therapist developed a plan just before the party. Jenny chose to avoid the punch and only drink what she could cope with. She consumed soft drinks, possessed no more than one alcoholic beverage, stayed no longer than just three hours, and ask her boyfriend to pick her up after the party.

Example 2

John believed he had been "no good" and a "failure" in the office, in his romantic relationship as well as in his immediate environment. Through time, he came to realize bad stuff would take place and that things could always be problematic for him. This made him give up easily and believe there is "no point in striving."

John's therapist helped him identify all these beliefs and considered evidence for and from them. He discovered that he viewed the world in black and white, and commenced challenging himself to find the balance. John also figured out how to be more assertive and also perform activities that made him feel good about himself.

Cognitive Tools

Once individuals tackle the practices of self-monitoring and personal examination, they often uncover dysfunctional methods of thinking and problematic ways of thinking which prohibit them from success. If and when you locate these achievement banning mental routines, you can alter them using the practice of cognitive restructuring, or the practice of determining, hard, and altering unwanted thoughts into more prudent choices. The dysfunctional imagined record and ABCD version we touched above will steer you toward discovering and transforming success banning cognitions.

Behavioral Tools

While trying to transform dysfunctional methods of thinking and problematic habits of the head there's an excellent strategy. CBT therapists may often have to help their sufferers find and release limiting core beliefs observed below surface degree cognitions. As it's improbable to triumph without needing complete confidence in ourselves, letting go of these unwanted beliefs we hold about ourselves is equally vital for achievement. Luckily, we've come across evidence that no longer serves our demands from job behavioral exercises and tasks. Behavioral stimulation (climbing good reinforcement & decreasing unfavorable behavioral routines), behavioral rehearsal (training for impending occasions & situations), along with behavioral experiments (information-gathering exercises used to test the validity of thoughts & beliefs) are three common behavioral tools.

360-degree opinions

If you wish to improve your levels of social-emotional skills, your abilities to communicate with others, along with your professional standing, one effective instrument is 360-degree feedback or multisource opinions. While 360-degree evaluations are most frequently utilized in settings that are professional, they can also be useful to gauge others view us in societal, family, and community surroundings. By having others that you regularly interact with fill out a test assessment of one's weakness and strengths, you can acquire invaluable insight into the ways others view you personally and discover undeveloped skills which could help elevate you to the next level. It is critical not to become up-set, as most of the feedback you receive needs to be accepted whole-heartedly and employed for expansion.

Values Clarification Exercise

The last tool we're going to look at that will be terrific for people strug-gling to locate meaning in existence is available from the shape of the popular Acceptance and Commitment Therapy clinic called the values caution practice. It's fairly easy to fault individual development with the faulty notion that success, money, and improved connections are the things we should be after. Reevaluate your values and determine the type of individual you wish to become. This may help steer you towards improving your levels of well-being.

Depending upon the verifiable efficacy of CBT, it is clear how all of us can utilize its orderly strategies to spiral towards the accomplishment of our goals. We could all achieve our goals by defining good results, building intelligent goals, committing to self-monitoring and self-eval-uation, while also employing CBT techniques to help along the way.

Chapter 4: CBT Advantages and Methods

In the present society, health practitioners and psychiatrists are speedy to prescribe psychotropic drugs which often accompany dangerous negative side effects for any disorder that is due to idea patterns. But if you were told that there was a superior, more secure way to take care of and cure strain and mind disorders through cognitive behavioral therapy, would you try it?

CBT is just a form of psychotherapy which highlights the importance of inherent thoughts in ascertaining how we act and feel. CBT is regarded as one of the absolute most prosperous forms of psychotherapy to emerge in decades; CBT has become the focus of countless scientific tests.

CBT therapists discover, investigate, and transform their particular thought patterns, and reactions since they are what creates our senses and determines our behaviors. Using CBT therapy boosts patient's quality of life and also help them handle stress better compared to patients battling with tough situations independently.

What may surprise you about CBT as a core basic theory is that extreme scenarios, interactions with different people, and negative events are not usually accountable for our poor moods and problems. Instead, CBT therapists view precisely the opposite as being the cause. It's our reactions to events, the more things we tell ourselves in regards to these occasions—that can be within our control—that wind up affecting our quality of life. This is great news because it indicates we can modify ourselves.

Using cognitive behavioral therapy, we can learn to alter the way we feel, which in turn alters the way we see and cope with tough circumstances when they arise. We are now better at intercepting disruptive notions that cause us to be stressed, isolated, and depressed, and likely too mentally obese and reluctant to change negative habits. When we could accurately and calmly start looking at situations without distorting reality or incorporating limitations or fears, we will be able to understand just how to react appropriately to help us feel better in the long run in a means that creates us feel speediest in the very long run.

Here are a few benefits of cognitive behavioral therapy:

1. Lowers Symptoms of Depression

CBT is one of the most rapid, empirically supported treatments for depression. Studies demonstrate that CBT helps patients overcome signs of depression: such rage and low drive. It also lowers their risk of relapses in the future. CBT is thought to get the job done well. It's known for relieving depression because it delivers changes in cognition (feelings) that fuels vicious cycles of unwanted feelings along with rumination.

An analysis published in the journal, Cognitive Behavioral Therapy for Mood Disorders found that CBT is protective towards severe episodes of depression and can be utilized alongside or in place of anti-depressant drugs. CBT has also demonstrated promise as an approach for helping handle post-partum depression as well as an adjunct to drug treatment for bipolar patients.

Also, preventative cognitive therapy (a version of CBT) paired with anti-depressants were found to help patients that underwent long-term depression. Even the 2018 human study analyzed 289 members and afterward randomly assigned them to PCT and antidepressants, anti-depressants independently, or PCT with diminishing use of anti-depressants after healing. The study found that clinical therapy coupled together with antidepressant treatment was first-rate in comparison to alcoholism treatment alone.

1. Reduces Anxiety

There are strong indications that CBT could cure transmitted illnesses. Strong signs are seeing CBT cure for illnesses that are transmitted, such as panic disorders, obsessive-compulsive disorder, social anxiety disorder, generalized anxiety disorder, and post-traumatic stress disorder pressure disease. Overall, CBT shows both effectiveness in randomized controlled trials and efficacy in both naturalistic settings between patients with anxiety and therapists. Researchers have found that CBT functions well as an organic treatment for anxiety because it comprises various combinations of the following techniques:

Psycho-education regarding the character of fear and anxiety, self-monitoring of outward symptoms, bodily exercises, cognitive restructuring (by way of instance disconfirmation), the image along with in vivo experience of feared stimuli (exposure therapy), weaning from unsuccessful safety signals, along with relapse prevention.

1. Helps Deal with Eating Disorders

CBT has been proven to help significantly handle the underlying psychopathology of eating disorders and question the over-evaluation of shape and weight. Besides, it can interfere with the aid of sterile body weights, improve urge control, help prevent binge eating or purging, decrease feelings of isolation, and also support patients eventually become comfortable with "trigger food items" or situations using exposure therapy. Cognitive therapy is now the procedure of choice in treating bulimia nervosa and "eating disorders not otherwise defined" (ED-NOS) the two most popular eating disease diagnoses. There's also evidence it could assist in healing around sixty percent of people with anorexia, which is considered to be one of the most challenging mental illnesses to cure or prevent from failing.

1. Reduce Addictive Behaviors and Substance Abuse

Studies have shown that CBT is excellent in supporting cannabis and other drug dependencies, such as alcohol and opioid addiction. It also helps people quit smoking tobacco and gambling. Studies published in the Oxford Journal of Medicine Public Health concerning solutions for smoking cessation have also found that working skills realized during CBT periods were tremendously helpful in cutting relapses in cigarette quitters and it appears to be superior to other curative approaches. There is also stronger support for CBT's behavioral procedures (assisting to stop impulses) at the treatment of problematic gaming addictions in comparison to control remedies.

1. Helps Improve Self-Esteem and Assurance

Even if you never suffer from any significant mental problems in any respect, CBT can assist you in replacing harmful, negative thoughts that cause low self-esteem, with positive affirmations and expectations. This helps open new tactics to handle stress, improve relationships, and increase the drive to try new issues.

1. Helps you become more rational

The brain essentially acts as a neutral object, giving a response based on the information at its disposal and also the way it was trained to respond. Cognitive therapy trains the brain to act rationally.

In CBT, it is believed that our thoughts lead to how we feel, behave and handle situations. The good thing about this is that we have a chance to change how we think and act right even if the situation remains unchanged.

CBT helps patients to control the thinking pattern that leads to irrational behaviors. Those undergoing CBT treatment are thought strategies with which they can cope better whenever automatic negative thoughts (ANTs) arise. CBT helps to develop ways to control the brain.

1. It boosts your self-belief

CBT helps to boost your self-confidence and works on your belief system, so you gain much better control of your thoughts. With self-confidence, you will be able to face any challenge that comes your way to achieving success and attaining your goals.

1. It helps you stay calm and relaxed

The initial stage of learning about social anxiety therapy is to devise a new way to anxiety response. With CBT treatment one won't be frightened by anxiety or anything that happens abruptly as we approach things with much peace and calmness. It teaches one best way to handle different kinds of situations that may arise in a more relaxed manner.

1. CBT helps to raise your expectations as you expect better outcomes

Due to our prior history and self-doubts, we often expect negative things to happen to us. We are always expecting things to turn out bad for us. CBT works on those thoughts and your belief system so that you can start acting more rational. As our thoughts and action become more rational, our expectations also turn out to be more logical as expert positive things to happen.

With CBT, we are made to repeatedly question ourselves to ascertain if our old beliefs are rational or not. Are they fact-based? Alternatively, are they things that have been our norm for years, and we have never questioned it? What is the real truth?

Do we pay attention to feedback from others or do we only pay attention to our internal negative conclusions? Is there any chance that we've fallen into the trap of self-brainwashing over the years?

Our own old automatic negative thoughts can reprocess through-out the brain. Have you found a way to stop them? Have you explored the possible explanation for your actions and have you thought about it that there might be no justifiable reason to feel fearful and anxious?

As our belief system is transformed by our thoughts and beliefs which bring about physical changes in the brain. An improved way of thinking leads us to expect a different outcome, a positive one. Your outcome depends on what you think about the outcome.

Other benefits of cognitive behavioral therapy include:

- Preventing the relapse of an addiction
- Resolving issues in relationships
- Recognizing negative thoughts and emotions
- Chronic pain management
- Anger Management
- Ability to coping with grief and loss
- Dealing with sleep disorders

How Cognitive Behavior Therapy Works

CBT operates by pinpointing thoughts that continuously arise us-ing them as signs for favorable activity and substituting them with healthy, and far more empowering alternatives.

The heart of CBT is mastering self-coping techniques, offering in-dividuals the ability to handle their reactions/responses of situations logically, alter the thoughts they tell themselves, and exercise "logical self-counseling." While this helps the CBT therapist/counselor and af-fected person build confidence and possess a great romantic relation-ship, the power lies in the individual's control. How willing a patient is ready to explore her or his thoughts, be open-minded, complete re-search assignments and clinic patience throughout the CBT course of action, can all determine how favorable CBT will be for these.

Features that make CBT an Effective Tool

Pragmatic method

CBT techniques and theory are predicated on rational thinking, which means they aim to spot and use these details. Even the "inductive technique" of CBT encourages individuals to examine their own beliefs and perceptions to see whether they are realistic. With CBT, there is an inherent premise that many behavioral and psychological responses are all learned.

With CBT therapists' help, patients realize that their long-held premises and hypotheses are partially wrong, which reduces unnecessary anxiety and suffering.

Feeling difficult or debilitating emotions: Most CBT therapists can help individuals learn to remain calm and clear-headed even if they are faced with unwanted scenarios. Learning to accept difficult feelings as "part of life" is crucial, and it can help prevent one from developing a bad habit. Usually, we become upset about our strong feelings and become more distressed. Instead of adding self-blame, rage, despair, or disappointment to already-tough feelings, CBT instructs sufferers to calmly accept a problem without making it even worse.

Questioning and expressing

Cognitive behavioral therapists typically ask patients lots of questions to help them gain a fresh and realistic perspective about the problem and also assist them to control how they feel.

Definite Agendas and Techniques

CBT is usually done in a succession of sessions that all possess a particular objective, concept, or technique that work together. Unlike a few other types of therapy, sessions are not exclusively for the therapist and individual to speak openly without an agenda on your mind. CBT therapists teach their customers the way to handle challenging thoughts and feelings by practicing particular techniques during sessions which may, later on, be implemented into life when they're most wanted.

Cognitive Behavioral Therapy vs. Other Types of Psychotherapy

CBT can be a sort of psychotherapy, which means that it calls for open discussion between patient and therapist. You may know about several other forms of psychotherapy and you're wondering what makes CBT stand out. Sometimes when there is an overlap between several types of psychotherapy, a therapist could use techniques from various psychotherapy approaches to assist patients in attaining their goals. For example, to help anyone with a phobia, CBT may be coupled together with exposure therapy.

How is CBT different From Other Popular Forms of Therapy?

The National Alliance on Mental Illness states how CBT Is Different from other popular forms of therapy:

CBT vs. Dialectical Behavior Therapy (DBT)

CBT and DBT and are most likely the most comparable curative approaches; nevertheless DBT depends heavily on validation or accepting uncomfortable thoughts, feelings, and behaviors. DBT therapists help individuals detect balance between acceptance and change from using applications like mindfulness guided meditation.

CBT vs. Exposure Therapy

Exposure therapy is a sort of cognitive behavioral therapy that's often utilized to treat eating disorders, phobias, and anti-inflammatory disease. It teaches individuals to practice calming strategies and little series of "exposures" to triggers (issues which are most dreaded) to become less concerned with the outcome.

CBT vs. Interpersonal Therapy

Social therapy concentrates on the relationships a patient has together with his or her family, friends, and co-workers. Focusing on societal interactions and recognizing negative patterns such as isolation, jealousy, blame, or aggression are part of therapy. CBT can be employed with social therapy to help reveal subjective beliefs and notions forcing negative behavior and supporting the others.

CBT Journal work

Journal work is the most important part of CBT; this might help you;

- Practice balanced and accurate self-talk.

- Learn how to change and control aberrations and thoughts.

- Use self-examinations to reflect and respond in healthy and better ways.

- Learn how you can properly comprehend and precisely assess emotional behaviors such as external situations and reactions.

- Through utilizing different methods it's possible to learn how you can live well and balanced with both your mind and body.

Once more, the duration of time a person spends in treatment is usually less compared to some other therapy. Also, note that CBT will not *cure* depression or other issues, but rather you will get measurable relief while improving your daily life.

Chapter 5: Disorders, Medical, and Emotional Issues CBT is Expected to Treat

CBT can be very useful for a lot of disorders, medical, and emotional problems. Some of the common ones will be discussed in detail in subsequent chapters. Here is a brief overview of some disorders you should expect CBT to treat.

Panic Disorders

CBT assists in targeting panic disorder by bringing the client to what he/she fears most, these exposure periods assist every individual in learning that they could also experience symptoms of being aroused without having to fear what comes next. Interceptive exercise gives room for every individual to face the sensations they get physically that comes along with panic. Example, Hyperventilation or bodily spinning can also be introduced during sessions to help induce lightheadedness or feelings of dizziness. With imaginary exposures, the therapist reads scripts that focus on an individual's fears during the sessions over and over again until there is a feeling that the personal fears have reduced to some extent.

With Vivo Exposure, the individual's fears can be drastically reduced, allowing them to avoid situations that might cause a panic attack. On certain occasions, there are groups of challenging problems that are brought about, and that individual follows the steps with the aid of the therapist. Afterwards, the individual's attitude will change, allowing them to consistently seek out and face every hard situation.

Depression

CBT can also help depression by using a known technique which is also known as behavior activation. Using the behavior activation, both the therapist and client work together to introduce new events that are pleasant to the individual's life. This will help to change the mood of that individual by avoiding the reverse, increasing self-confidence, increasing the level of usefulness, physical activity, and ultimately reducing negative thoughts. Behavior activation contains many different behaviors, the ones that are most common are the ones that bring out more pleasant activities, and other behaviors that will stress out the individuals like cleaning a messy apartment, calling alienated family members, or filing taxes.

Attention Deficit/Hyperactivity Disorder (ADHD)

Under normal conditions, treatment for the first line of ADHD is medications (psychostimulants). Most times, only medications aren't enough for many people who have ADHD. CBT for ADHD aims to assists many individuals in changing coping skills to handle their symptoms and deal with functional and emotional effects that comes with people living with the disorder. Patients are always encouraged to give real-life examples of some specific issues and difficulties they face with the therapist to help find the best solution. It is also important that the therapist and patient introduce some problems that might end up arising and make plans that will help solve them.

Obsessive Compulsive Disorder (OCD)

The preferred method for today's treatment for OCD is weekly CBT treatment that usually involves (exposure and response/ritual prevention) ERP exercise. Exposure and response prevention connote that the first individual introduces themselves to thoughts, objects, images, and situations that make them anxious or obsessed (exposure). Individuals then oppose doing a compulsive behavior when the obsessions or anxiety is triggered that is response prevention. This helps stop or reduce compulsions.

Social Phobia/Social Anxiety

The therapist that uses CBT to assist clients in getting a new way of behaving and thinking by adopting realistic and positive thoughts to change all bad and unrealistic thoughts. Cognitive restructuring is necessary for those individuals that are faced with societal anxiety, as they are learning to question and challenge every truth behind their beliefs. This can be done by giving solid evidence against every other belief that is problematic in a Socratic conversation. Behavioral experiments are also important as they show individuals that disastrous events known by irrational beliefs don't always end up happening during the periods of exposure exercises. This helps explain lies about their beliefs.

Bipolar Disorder

Certainly, most of the patients that are suffering from Bipolar disorder are being given medications, most of the time mood stabilizers, and initial evidence explains to us that CBT is an effective therapy to pharmacotherapy. CBT for Bipolar disorder exerts more force on mood regulations and psycho-education. Psycho-education helps to educate individuals on what the illness is all about and the consequences, their side effects, medication options, symptoms, as well as the early warning signs of episodes. CBT helps individuals to track and also identify their mood swings and decrease emotional reactivity through mindful exercise, breathing, or self-soothing (distractions).

Generalized Anxiety Disorder (GAD)

CBT is very effective in treating GAD; it helps decrease not just the actual symptoms of anxiety, but also what is associated with depressive symptoms, which will improve quality of life. One of the most effective trainings for GAD is what is known as relaxation training. During sessions, individuals must learn how to reduce the tension in the muscle and shallow breathing, as they are both known to cause anxiety and stress. The two strategies that are commonly used in CBT are paced respiration, which involves being aware of reducing your breath and progressive muscle relaxation which systematically involves tension and relaxation of different muscle groups. There are other useful relaxation methods that can be used which include; meditation, listening to music, massage, and yoga.

Schizophrenia

CBT has now been recommended as a treatment to be used for schizophrenia, it can be used alongside medications. Using CBT, the individuals get to know that there is a link that connects their feelings and patterns of thinking that underlies their discomfort. It also focuses on disputing and identifying the client's irrational beliefs through behavioral experiments and certain discoveries.

CBT can be useful in helping the clients in every aspect so they can validate their beliefs. These kinds of experiment usually encourage clients to be active which eventually leads to a deeper level understanding.

Bulimia Nervosa

CBT is the most used treatment procedure for bulimia; the illness at its core has concerns with the shape of the body and weight, which leads to excessive dieting and behaviors that are controlled by body image.

Excessive dieting also makes one susceptible to rapid eating; CBT treatment focuses on improving the motivation to change, change dieting to a flexible and regular one, and reduce your concerns about weight, preventing relapse and body shape. CBT has also shown to be more efficient and acceptable antidepressant medications in destroying excessive eating, CBT is expected to remove excess eating and purging in almost 30-50% cases and this decreases the level of other psychiatric symptoms and improves social functioning and self-esteem.

Fear of Flying/Flying phobia

CBT is also very effective for the treatment of many phobias, the flight phobia is a very common complaint that CBT can efficiently treat. Psycho-education is one of the most important components used in CBT treatment, and this is usually added with cognitive training and relaxation techniques. Imaginal exposure is also very useful; it can assist clients in thinking about situations where the clients are on a plane, or any other circumstance that might help induce fear, this will try to raise their anxiety over a short period. However, once they are thinking about the same thing over and over again, their anxiousness decreases each time and this will help them handle much deeper real-life situations much better. Recent development in treating the phobia of flying is reality exposure where individuals are exposed to their fears in a 3D computer-compilation. This will help create a real-life environment, the same principle of being exposed technically works the same.

There are several other disorders that CBT can be used for; we will also discuss some of them in details in the ensuing chapters.

Chapter 6: CBT for Depression

Life could be funny at times; and sometimes, you feel like you are down. When you are down or you think that life is against you is what every other person feels in today's world. Over 14.8 million adults in the US are affected by a Major Depressive Disorder according to the Anxiety and Depression Association of America.

Depression can be serious as it gives room for a "normal" functioning difficulty which means so much that you simply get through the day by totally being overwhelmed, and then you can turn to alcohols and drugs for more comfort. When you are down, it is like the world is crashing down, just know that there is a way out and there is no need for you to keep suffering.

CBT for depression starts with placing greater attention on reducing the symptoms of depression through cognitive and behavioral techniques intended to detect and challenge harmful automatic thoughts.

Once there has been a significant reduction in the symptom of depression, individuals practicing CBT may then be able to focus on how they can prevent future occurrence.

Cognitive Behavioral therapy for people who are depressed can help restore the zeal you have for the world we are living in; it can assist you in thinking in a more healthy way, help to prevail over an addiction. Before going into details of what CBT is, and how it can help to treat depression, though, it is very important to know the primary types of depression.

Types of Depression

Persistent Depressive Disorder (PDD)

This is also formerly known as dysthymia; it is a type of depression that most times continues for two years. Generally, this is much more severe than even major depression, but you will experience similar symptoms. PDD also shows itself as stress, inability to enjoy life, and irritability.

Major Depression

This involves suffering from depressive symptoms (5 or more) for about two weeks; major depressive episodes are disabling. It might interfere with the ability for you to work, sleep, eat, and study. These kinds of episodes only happen for a few periods throughout your lifetime, after a terrible experience like the demise of a family member or the downfall of any relationship.

Bipolar Depression

This type of depressive disorder shows when your life is in a period of shifting mood cycles that includes harsh or gentle high (hypomania or mania) depressive lows and crushing.

Now you are already aware of the major types of depression disorders, how common it might be, the symptoms; it is good to know that there is an effective treatment for depression. CBT is one of the types of psychotherapy that changes your thought pattern; it also assists in changing your moods and behaviors. The therapy originates from the work of Aaron T.Beck and Albert Ellis in 1950-1960s. Generally speaking, CBD is a treatment for depression that blends cognitive and behavioral therapy in which the therapist assists in identifying a particular bad pattern, and your behaviors response to stress, and challenging circumstances.

Signs and Symptoms of Depression

If you have a concern about depression, ask yourself these questions whether you will be able to identify with any of the following symptoms:

- Lack of interest in things you usually enjoy

- Uncontrollable negative thoughts

- Irritability, short-tempered, and aggression

- Engaging in reckless behavior

- Feelings of helplessness and hopelessness

- Appetite changes, such as eating far less or too much

- Self-loathing; a feeling of being worthless and guilty

- Using illegal or prescription drugs in excess

- Unnatural tiredness

- Drinking more alcohol than usual

- Unexplained pains and aches which also includes stomach pains, back pains, sore muscles, and headaches.

If you answer to any or more of these, you might be depressed, and Cognitive Behavioral therapy might be able to help.

Going for a CBT depression can be discouraging. However, here is a little guide of what will be involved, so be prepared:

Therapy

You may want to meet with your therapist for a period of 5 to 20 weekly or biweekly periods. In general, periods might last between 30 to 60 minutes, all through the beginning of 2-4 sessions; your therapist will know if you are truly right for the treatment or whether you are comfortable with it. A therapist can ask about your background or your past, CBT also focuses on what the present is all about, but at times, it can be imperative to open up about your past and how it affects you presently. You decide what exactly you need and how well you want to deal with it, along with your therapist.

The work

With the support of your therapist, each problem you have is broken down into different parts. To help you with that, you might be asked to keep a diary to assist you in identifying every one of your emotions, personal ways, and physical feelings. Both of you take a look at the behaviors, thoughts, and feelings to see how they are affecting each other and how they might also affect you. If they are not realistic or helpful; your therapist might figure out a way to change any negativity. The therapist might also give you "assignments" which involves practicing how to identify changes you will need to make every day in your life. During the time of every meeting, you will have more opportunities to talk about your progress since the last meeting; if there is a specific duty that is not working out for you, you should discuss such issues. You might never be able to do things that you love to do; you might also dictate the pace of your therapy and can also keep developing your skills when the sessions are complete. This will allow you to remain happy for many years to come.

How Does Cognitive Behavioral Therapy (CBT) Differ From Other Depression Treatments?

The method and general focus of Cognitive Behavioral Therapy is kind of different from many other, more traditional depression treatments. For instance, Cognitive Behavioral Therapy: Modifies behaviors in the immediate present while changing your thought patterns.

CBT majorly addresses your problematic thinking and undesirable behaviors.

• Clear goals are fixed for each session and the long-term. i.e., Goal-oriented.

• CBT is educational. You monitor your thoughts and feelings, and then you commit these to paper. The therapist will also teach you essential coping skills, such as problem-solving.

• Makes you play an active part in your learning and recovery. You will also be able to complete "homework" assignments that are reviewed at the beginning of the next session.

• CBT employs multiple strategies, including role-playing, guided discovery and behavioral experiments.

• CBT is time limited.

How Cognitive Behavioral Therapy Can Help With Depression

We are all aware of how debilitating depression can be. Depression is an extremely common condition. The illness impacts your life negatively as well as the lives of your family and friends. It can go a long way to affect your employers and co-workers.

Depression has impacted negatively on the general functioning of the society as a whole. For example, it is a fact that the illness imposes a financial burden on you, the sufferer, as well as on your family, caregiver, your employer, and insurance provider.

CBT can guarantee a new lease on life if you're going through depression. Conversely, if you have severe major depression, CBT, delivered in conjunction with other medication, is a very effective or efficient treatment.

Thinking negatively can slow depression recovery, and the reason is self-evident: If you have negative thoughts, you're more likely to stay depressed. But what is less obvious is the way people with depression deal with their positive emotions. Researchers have made an astounding observation: People with depression never lack positive emotions; they will never allow themselves to feel them.

This cognitive style is known as "dampening," and it involves suppressing positive emotions with thoughts such as, "This good feeling won't last." "I don't deserve to be this happy." For example, a new mom with postpartum depression might begin to doubt herself and ability to recover because she's a bad mother for being depressed in the first place.

Defensive pessimism makes people with depression think this way. It seeks to protect against getting high hopes dashed. "You never want to be the fool, so you resort to dampening positive thoughts to protect yourself from potential disappointment."

CBT is believed to help significantly with depression treatment. With CBT, you and your therapist work hand to hand, i.e., together, to reach an agreement on behavior patterns that need to be changed. The purpose or goal is to recalibrate the part of your brain that's keeping such a tight hold on happy thoughts.

An unanticipated reaction to a major life events might be at the root of the dampening effect. Through CBT, you and your therapist address it and work toward putting it into perspective.

Regular Cognitive Behavior therapy sessions and work people do on there can help to reinforce the new patterns. Recognizing those negative thoughts and leaving them behind can be very liberating.

Cognitive Behavioral Therapy Techniques to Counteract the Negative Thinking of Depression

People with depression don't respond well to self-study. For this reason, it's recommended to commit to CBT for at least seven weeks. Your therapist will teach you strategies that can help frustrate or counteract the negative thinking associated with depression. He or she can also help you stay on track with practicing the techniques.

Here is the list of CBT strategies you might work on with your therapist:

1. Locate the problem and brainstorm or investigate solutions.

Talking and Journaling with your therapist can help you discover the root of your depression. Once you have any idea or impression, write down what's bothering you and think of ways to improve the situation.

A hallmark of depression is hopelessness — not believing that things can ever get better. Write down lists of things that can be done to improve a situation and it will help to ease depressive feelings. For instance, if you're battling loneliness, action steps may involve joining a local club in line with your interests or signing up for dating online.

1. Write self-statements to counteract negative thoughts.

After finding the root problems of your depression, think of all the negative thoughts you use to dampen positive ones. Write a self-statement to counteract with each negative thought. Always note your self-statements and repeat them back to yourself when you notice the little voice in your head creeping in to snuff out a positive thought. Soon enough, you'll create new associations, replacing all the negative thoughts with positive ones.

1. Self-affirmations shouldn't be overly positive or else the mind might find it difficult to accept it.

For instance, if the negative thought says, "I feel so depressed right now," instead of saying, "I'm feeling really happy now," it could be better rephrased as, "Every life experience ups and downs, and mine does, too." This tells you that it's okay to bump up the degree or rate of happiness you experience. At the same time, one's mind applauds itself for keeping joy and happiness in check to protect from disappointment. It's very good to recognize that part of you that's trying to do something healthy.

At some point, self-statements become too routine and need to be refreshed. Rephrase your self-statements or translate it into any language that you speak, perhaps it could spring up your happy feelings a bit. For instance, the self-statement, "It's very good to explore my ups" might become "It's good to have a very super 'up' day."

If you have a partner or loved one suffering from depression, there is a possibility that CBT will effectively treat them depending on the severity. Also, you might face the challenge about your loved one feeling reluctant to seek help for depression.

The ideal way to raise such person's spirits toward going for CBT session is to calmly discuss their fears and concerns about going for the session, instead of telling them they have to go. Show concern and support and reassure them that you don't think something is wrong with them; instead, you only want them to get some help to cope with their present challenge.

Sometimes, depressed people want help but don't have an idea about what to do and where to start. By offering to assist in visiting a therapist to schedule an appointment can improve their chances of committing to CBT.

Chapter 7: CBT for Anxiety

CBT is mostly used everywhere as therapy for anxiety disorders; many researches have been undergone to show that the effectiveness of this treatment of phobia's, generalized disorders, and panic disorder among so many other likely conditions. This examines the terrible patterns and aberrations in the way we view things like the world and ourselves generally, just as the name implies, it involves two categories;

1. **Behavior Therapy:** This looks deeply into how you can react and behave in circumstances that bring about anxiety.
2. **Cognitive Therapy:** This observes how bad thoughts or cognitions add to the anxiety.

The fundamental proposition of CBT is that our thoughts and not what happens externally affect how we are feeling, i.e., not exactly the circumstance that you are feeling right now that determines the perception of that particular situation. Example, Let's just say that you have been invited somewhere for a party. Let's look at how well you have different ways of viewing the invitation and how this thought can affect your emotional state.

Situation 1: A friend gives you an invitation to a big party

Thought A: The party sounds like there will be lots of fun, I'm excited to get out and meet new people.

Emotions: Tranquility, excitement.

Thoughts B: Parties are not my kind of thing, I prefer to stay in and watch movies.

Emotions: Neutral.

Thoughts C: I do not know what to say or how to act when I am at a party, I will probably make a fool of myself if I go.

Emotions: Unhappy, Anxious.

Now you know that one type of event can turn out different for people with different types of emotions. It all strongly depends on every individuals' expectations, beliefs, and attitude. For this type of people with anxiety disorders, terrible patterns of thinking evoke the terrible beliefs and thoughts. This conception is brought about when you change your way you think, and you can also change the way you feel.

Cognitive Behavioral Techniques you will need to beat anxiety

1. The Ability to Recognize Rumination

Rumination is when you are bothered over and over again by a worrisome thought when you think about issues; it lowers your capacity to solve any problems. If you are constantly ruminating, it is best to patiently wait to solve the problem first until when you discover that the problem has gone beyond the issue of solving and then begin to ruminate over it.

If you can learn to recognize when you are ruminating, then it is proper for you to use Cognitive Behavioral methods or being mindful to assist you in stopping the act of ruminating. The right thing to do when ruminating is to accept that you are having whatsoever thought you have right now, know that you might not be accurate, but it allows those thoughts to quickly pass in their own time instead of blocking it away.

1. The Ability and Willingness to use Mindful Techniques

Mindful techniques also assist in decreasing anxiety and then raising your willpower, practicing being mindful will assist you in reducing avoidance, make other better choice even when the feelings are anxious, and this will help you reduce rumination. Try the 10-minute mindful walking exercise.

1. The Ability to Tolerate Uncertainty

Research has made it known that not enduring uncertainty is one of the significant factors in anxiety and being depressed. Not enduring uncertainty is having anxiety and when you are not 100% sure that a negative event will not happen. People who are not able to tolerate uncertainties often keep away from situations like reassurance seek, delay taking action, refusing to delegate, do excessive checking and procrastination.

1. Ability to Recognize Thoughts Distortions

Different types of thought aberrations include lowering your own personal ability to cope, personalized mind reading, being judgmental about other people or yourself, making too much of a negative forecast, every other person as white or black instead of gray, entitlement thoughts (example, thinking about the normal rules that should not apply) and many more. The major key is to know that thought aberration is to question yourself whenever you have the feelings of depression. You can also try doing a CBT Thought Record.

1. The Ability to Talk to Yourself, Kindly about your Imperfections and Mistakes

Criticizing yourself when you try something and make a mistake, or when your imperfections show up can likely lead to rumination and avoid coping. Studies have shown us that when you talk to yourself, it does not just make you feel better but also increase your self-esteem and improves motivation.

Thoughts challenging in CBT for anxiety

The cognitive restructuring is also known as thought challenging is a series of steps that help to confront the bad thinking ways that most of the time contributes to your anxiety and then change them with more realistic, positive thoughts. This takes about three steps;

• Replacing Negative Thoughts with Realistic Thoughts

Once you know the irrational and negative aberrations in your thoughts, you can then change them with fresh and positive thoughts. Your therapist can devise a calming and realistic statement that you can always tell yourself when you are preventing or facing a circumstance that increases your anxiety level.

• Identifying your Negative Thoughts

With anxiety disorders, some situations are known to be very deadly than they are known to be, to someone with a phobia for germs, shaking someone's else hands may seem threatening. Although it might be possible for you to see that it's an irrational fear, knowing your personal irrational, fearful thoughts can be very hard. One way is to question yourself about what you are thinking about when you are anxious. Your personal therapist can assist you with this process.

• Challenging your Negative Thoughts

Using this method, your therapist can help you acquire how to examine anxiety-provoking thoughts; this also involves asking about the facts for your threatening thoughts, testing out the truth about the negative forecast, and analyzing beliefs that are not helping. Methods used for challenging negative thoughts involves weighing the pros and cons of worrying, conducting experiments, or keeping away from the things that you fear and know the realistic chance that you have been anxious about will suddenly happen.

To know how these challenging thoughts work during CCBT, understand the following example; Maria will not take the subway just because she is scared she might pass out and then people might think she is actually crazy. Her therapist told her to jot down her terrible thoughts, the cognitive aberrations, or identifying what the error is in whatever she thinks about and then come up with an interpretation that is rational. The outcomes are stated below;

Challenging Negative Thoughts

Negative thought A: What if I pass out in the subway?

Cognitive aberrations: Forecast the worst.

More realistic thoughts: I have never passed out before, so it is not certain that I will.

Negative thought B: Once I pass out, it is going to be bad.

Cognitive aberration: Blowing things out of proportion

More Realistic Thoughts: If I pass out, I come around in a few minutes. That will be so terrible.

Negative thoughts C: People might assume that I am crazy

Cognitive Aberrations: Jump to conclusions

More realistic thoughts: People are most likely to be more concerned if I am okay.

Change negative thoughts with more represented one is much easier than done. Often, bad thoughts are part of lifelong ways of thinking; it involves doing extra work to break that habit. That is one of the reasons why CBT involves you practicing alone and at home too. CBT also involves;

• Confronting your fears (either in real life or imaginary).

• Learn to know when you are already feeling anxious and what that feels like in the body.

• Learn to cope with skills and relaxation methods to counteract pain and anxiety.

Exposure Therapy for Anxiety

Anxiety is not a favorable experience, so it is best naturally to keep away
if you can, one of the methods that most people use is by staying clear
of those problems that make them feel anxious. If you have fears for
heights, you might try to drive hours out of your way to avoid crossing
a very tall bridge, or if the fear of public speaking gets your stomach in
knots, you might as well skip your best friend's wedding just to avoid
making a toast. Aside from the fact that it might not be convenient,
you will not have the opportunity of overcoming them.

Exposure therapy, as the name, implies that vulnerability to circumstances or objects that you tend to fear, the conception is that
through consistent vulnerability, you will be able to feel a soaring control sense over every circumstance and then the anxiety begins to reduce. The exposure can be done in any of the two ways; you might want
to imagine a scary problem for you to face a real-life situation. Exposure
therapy might be used alone, or it might be used as part of the conduct-
ed CBT.

Systematic Desensitization

Instead of facing your greatest fear immediately, which can be used
in exposure therapy, traumatizing which usually begins with problems
that are only gentle threatening and this works up from there. This
stepwise method is also known as systematic desensitization allows you
to gradually replace your confidence, challenge your fears, and master
skills to influence his panic.

Facing the fear of flying
Step A: Check out the photos of planes
Step B: Watch videos of planes on a flight

Step C: Watch how real planes take off

Step D: Book a plane ticket

Step E: Pack for your flight

Step F: Drive to airport

Step G: Check-in for your flight

Step H: Wait to board

Step I: Get on the plane

Step J: Take the flight.

Systematic desensitization involves three parts;

Learning Relaxation Skills

First of all, your personal therapist will explain to you a relaxation method which includes deep breathing or muscle relaxation which you can practice alone at home or in the therapy. Immediately, you start facing your fears, and this relaxation method will assist you in decreasing your physical anxiety response (like hyperventilating and trembling) also to encourage relaxation.

Creating a Step-By-Step List

The next agenda is to create a list of 10-20 scary circumstances that might increase your final goal, example, if one of your final goals is to face your fear of flying, you could solve this by simply taking a look at photos of planes and ending it with an actual flight. Each step should be as actual practical as possible, with a measurable and clear objective.

Working Through the Steps

Under the process of your therapist, you will start to work through the list to stay in each scary circumstance until your fears are gone, that way you will learn to know that your feelings might not hurt you and they will not leave, every time anxiety gets too extreme, you will learn to move to the relaxation technique that is learned. Immediately, you have been relaxed again, you can turn the attention back to the situation, in this way, you will work through the methods till you have been able to finish every step without feeling totally discomforted.

Complementary Therapies for Anxiety Disorder

As you begin to examine your personal anxiety disorder in therapy, you might also want to fully experiment with other complementary therapies that are intended to bring down your stress level by assisting you in achieving balance emotionally.

- Relaxation methods such as medication that is mindful, progressive muscle relaxation that can be regularly practiced and can decrease anxiety, increase your emotional well-being.

- Hypnosis can be sometimes used together with CBT for anxiety even when you are in a state of constant, profound relaxation; hypnotherapist uses various therapeutic methods to assist you in confronting your fears and looking at them from another angle.

- Exercise is one of the natural anxiety relievers and also increase stress, research has made it known that even a little period of exercise for about 30 minutes 3-5 times in a week can also provide better relief for anxiety. To achieve a better result, a maximum of an hour of exercise will do on most occasions.

- Biofeedback makes use of sensors that aid specific physiological functions like breathing, muscle tension, and heart rate which is used to explain to you how your body responds to anxiety and learn to control it using relaxation methods.

Making Anxiety Therapy Work for You

You cannot quickly rush to fix anxiety disorders, to overcome anxiety really takes being committed to it, and also take lots of time. Therapy also includes confronting your fears rather than staying away from them, at times, most people feel worse even before they get better. The most necessary thing is to get used to treatment and follow the advice that is given to you by your therapist. If you are discouraged with the way at which you are recovering, just keep it in the back of your mind that the therapy given for anxiety is always very efficient, and you will surely get the gains if you are able to see it through.

You can also give full support to your own anxiety therapist by always making good choices, everything you do from your level of activities to your life socially affects how anxious you become. Always set the pace for success by making an effort to allow relaxation, positive mental outlook and even vitality in your life daily.

- Adopt a lifestyle that is healthy, physical activities when done totally reduces anxiety and tension, so you should create time for regular exercises. Make sure you do not use drugs or alcohols to work with the symptoms and try to keep away from stimulants like nicotine or caffeine which allows for anxiety disorders to worsen.

- Learn about anxiety: For you to be able to overcome anxiety, it is very important that you learn to know where the problem lies and that is really where education lies, just know that only education will not completely cure an anxiety disorder, but it will assist you in getting more out of the therapy.

- Totally reduce stress in your life, and try to observe your life during stress, and look for methods to reduce it. Keep away from people who are always making you anxious and bluntly disagree on every responsibility, make extra time to have fun and have add relaxation to your daily schedule.

• Cultivate having the right connections with every other person, being lonely and isolation makes it very easy to become anxious. Reduce your exposure by reaching out to people, make it important to see your friends, join support groups and share your concerns and worries with your loved ones.

Chapter 8: CBT for Fear and Phobias

Certain people immediately form a negative mindset against others rather than encouraging themselves to get to know positive things about other people.

Buddying up with other person working on the same methods with you and your friends can be very exciting whenever you have a positive mind and experiences that you are sharing every day. Here are few ways to use CBT to eliminate fear and phobia.

1. Accept disappointment as a common part of life

Some unexpected circumstance is an aspect of life and how well you respond to it shows how quickly you will move forward. Some people might just be going through break up, and then begin to blame themselves for what happened. Thoughts such as "what good is it to look good? I will never meet someone else like him/her," is an example.

Action plan:

Try as much as possible to know that those scenarios can be out of your control

Work on those things that are within your reach write down the things that happened, the experience gained from it and things you hope you will be able to do differently another time, watch for bad thoughts always coming to your minds. This will guide you on how to move on and feel good about it.

1. End each day by visualizing the best part

When the day is over, note down or type into a journal the things in your life that you are always grateful for, record every positive thought. You could even share your thought online; this will help you find new friends or show you better ways to do things.

Treatment for Phobias

Phobias do not need to be treated until their fear is preventing them from performing the necessary task, working or having good relationships. Example, if you decide to live in the United States and you know that you have fears of tigers, you could decide not to visit the zoo; rather, you should spend more time learning how to treat your phobias. Most types of anxiety disorders have cures; showing that not all single treatment can work for all type of phobia. When you are looking for the treatment for a particular type of phobia, the methods each therapist might use may differ. Here are some common forms of therapy to treat phobias.

Cognitive Behavioral Therapies for Phobia's

Cognitive Behavioral Therapy (CBT) allows you to take charge of your fears by helping you gradually to change the way you think; its fundamental basis is the connections between thoughts, behaviors, and beliefs. A person who has phobia knows that his or her feared circumstances are really dangerous. It will then lead such person to develop negative thoughts as soon as such fear is faced. This might lead to several patterns to change his or her thoughts.

To successfully overcome this, the therapist might be needed first to develop a treatment plan. For instance, if you have a fear of dogs the treatment plan could be first to take out time to read all about dogs to watching movies about dogs. Also, take such person to a place where dogs are being taken care of to show that they are not harmful.

Group Therapies to Ease Fears

Cognitive Behavior theory is a very common type of groups that make up the phobia therapy, although, there are various forms of therapy to be used in this method. Some CBT sessions for phobia might be in the form of a seminar which may last for 1 hour or several days. For instance, those with the phobia of height or flying can assemble at the airport hotel for a brief meeting during the weekend. In this meeting, they will be able to engage themselves in combinations of vulnerability sessions and psych educational class within the airport.

Individual Therapy

Individual therapy makes it possible for the therapist and the individual to focus properly on each other, building a solid friendship and helping to work together to solve the issue. However, related therapies and psychoanalysis might progress for months or even many years while short-term therapies like CBT can produce results in just very few sessions.

Family Therapy

If the therapist discovers that the family could also contribute to the development of having phobias, it is possible to suggest the family as part of the therapy plans. A very common example is the application of the family therapy which allows for communications between other family members. Family therapy is a very common plan for children that have phobias.

Chapter 9: CBT for Maladaptive or Bad Habits

Maladaptive Behaviors refers to those behaviors that refrain your ability to improve to specific healthy situations. They prevent you from coping with the demands and stress associated with life. Often, they are used to stop anxiousness; maladaptive behaviors lead to non-productive and dysfunctional results in which they are more harmful than they are helpful. Maladaptive Behaviors can be grouped as dysfunctional since they give short-term assistance from discomfort and they do not cope with anxiety for a while. These behaviors are not productive as they are not doing anything0 to prevent the problem and this may serve as the strength of an underlying difficulty.

Some known maladaptive behaviors interact with panic disorder, and they include:

Avoidance

For so many people, the symptoms they get from panic disorder often provokes avoidance behavior. This can lead to agoraphobia, which is a common complication that happens in 25%-50% of people with panic disorder. Agoraphobia takes little time to unfold or can come on quickly. Some of the people suffering believe that the symptom of agoraphobia takes place immediately after their first panic attack. Immediately it takes roots; avoidance behaviors multiply quickly.

Substance Misuse

People, who have an anxiety disorder which also includes the agoraphobia and panic disorder, often use alcohol or other substance as a method of coping with anxiety and fears.

Research has shown that people who have an anxiety disorder are more likely to have substance abuse or alcohol abuse disorder than those who do not have an anxiety disorder. Abusing alcohol or other forms of drugs to control anxiety and stress is grouped as a maladaptive behavior because it provides only little relief from anxiety and this might create many more problems. Substance abuse does not fix any difficulty nor do long-term alcohol; drug abuse can lead to dependence, tolerance and for some people, addiction.

Withdrawing

Many life challenges do not need ongoing actions both mentally and behaviorally; often, we struggle and achieve success, there are also times that we struggle and yet still fail. When the latter occurs, it is possible to try again or get withdrawn from conflicts with the acceptance of our situations. When it comes to other anxiety or panic disorders, withdrawing is not attuned with recovery. This is a maladaptive behavior because it means we are going to succumb to the sickness and then not able to meet up with life's challenges. In reality, withdrawing means giving up!

Converting Anxiety to Anger

It is natural for those who are dealing with agoraphobia, panic disorder or another disorder to get frustrated easily due to their conditions. At times, this frustration leads to anger about yourself, anger towards people, and anger at what you are going through presently.

This type of anger exists in anxiety, and it's likened to a strong feeling that is natural in human experience. Everyone has felt angry at one point or another and getting angry is not exactly a bad thing. But, whenever you experience anger unhealthily, it becomes an issue with the fact that anger has a way of increasing your anxiety and makes your panic symptoms much worse. One interesting thing is that CBT works to manage your anger and assist you in finding ways to adapt to your anxiety.

Chapter 10: CBT for Obsession and OCD

A large database verifies the efficiency of CBT for treating OCD using E/RP. Methodologically, trials that are controlled for CBT in children and adults reported that the rate of success got to 85% (SOR: A). What qualified success, is that most of the patients responded positively to CBT, even if the symptoms remain, and there is a total cure, there might not be complete cleansing.

CBT is unlike other psychotherapies. Sadly, the total number of mental health professionals that are qualified and trained in CBT for OCD is very limited, which also includes having general information about the methods. The Obsessive-Compulsive Foundation records about 5 million Americans that have OCD lack means to behavioral therapy. Many patients that are seen in clinics have gone through traditional (talk therapies) or psychodynamics that are verified by little evidence. Such methods have the strength of recommendations (SOR) of C. As a result of this, many distressed individuals get incomplete treatment that includes medications or non-CBT psychotherapy.

Three aspects of CBT therapy for OCD

1. **Response prevention:** Preventing compulsive behaviors or ritualistic that might serve to decrease or keep away anxiety.
2. **Cognitive therapy:** Training every patient to know and avoid anxiety-provoking cognitions.
3. **Exposure:** Place the patients' circumstance that will bring about anxiety that is related to obsessions. Exposure is just for the patient to be able to confront their fears and decrease their response to anxiety.

Response Prevention

This involves you advising the patient to desist from engaging in the same continuous practices, or compulsions that are time consuming. This part is fundamentally based on the belief that rituals serve to decrease anxiety and therefore are reinforcing. Normally, E/RP is anxiety provoking for most patients, and as a result of this, it may be important to let them know that a feared circumstance will be given in an approach that is hierarchical, beginning with much easier things before moving to something harder. Once you complete the E/RP tasks guides' patient that the consequence of fears is not going to occur.

Cognitive Therapy

This takes into accounts that patients that have OCD have a different thought that is known to lead to the contribution and development and maintaining of their condition. There is a common theme that is specified within the population which includes the risk appraisal, example, "chance at which a house is burned with a cigarette is 25%."

An increased attitude for responsibility in spite of harm, example "I know the consequences of contracting HIV from using a public toilet are very slim, but I cannot be sure that I won't contract it." OCD in most adults has also been related to the way of thought-action fusion in which bad actions and thoughts are seen as synonyms. Such non-adaptive cognitive steps often make compulsive behavior, and patients with less OCD can cope with bad thoughts, the cognitive part of CBT address the issues behind it and exposes patient's ways to improve their thinking.

Exposure

Also, when the family is involved is always known to be central to the success of CBT. Family members can also help in accommodating the patients' symptoms by encouraging avoidance, inadvertently precede the growth of the disorder by taking part in rituals (example, allowing compulsive avoidance of frightened stimuli, and allow delays that are associated with completion of ritual). Taking into account,

CBT at times, gives room for the parents, patient's spouse, and other significant people.

OCD Steps

Obsessive-Compulsive Disorder brings itself in many forms, and this surely goes beyond the common misconceptions that OCD is just like a small hand wash or checking light switch. Even though, there are well-grounded OCD compulsions like perceptions that fail to acknowledge the discomforting thoughts that come before Behaviors like that which might also fail to emphasize the harm the constant compulsion can cause.

There are many types of OCD capable of improving ones thought on any issue, fear or person, and often fixes the important issues in one's life. It can improve the thought on any subject, on any fear, on any person, and often fixes what is important in someone's life. Example, if you take religion very significant, OCD fixate on random disturbing thoughts that surround religion or making the person suffering know that their thoughts or actions will offend their God. Another example given is someone who starts a new relationship, OCD makes people question their sexuality, their feelings which results in constant rumination, while the person suffering may worry that they might mislead their partners.

Though there are so many forms of OCD; it has been known that somebody's OCD will be in one of the five main steps, with themes that often extend over between the steps too.

1. Contamination/ Mental Contamination
2. Symmetry and Ordering
3. Checking
4. Hoarding
5. Ruminations/Intrusive Thoughts

Hoarding

Hoarding is also included in the list and might be an OCD compulsion if it is known for a known obsessive reason. Nevertheless, some parts of hoarding are no longer taken to be OCD and might have separate condition together; we are looking at more hoarding-related disorders.

Another form of obsession known to be included in OCD is the inefficiency to remove bad or worn out possessions, also known as 'hoarding.' Hoarding, long known to be a type of Obsessive-Compulsive Disorder was correctly reclassified in 2013 journal of DSM-5 as an uncommon condition. However, it has become complicated because there are people with Obsessive-Compulsive Disorder will hoard for particular obsessive fears or worries and can still be diagnosed with OCD instead of hoarding disorder.

Checking

There is a need to check the compulsion, but the obsessive phobia might be to remove damage, leaks, harm, or fire. Common obsessive worries and compulsions include:

- Memories
- House/office alarm
- Water taps
- Reassurance
- Gas or electric stove knobs
- Car
- Door locks and or windows
- Emails or letters
- House lights and candles
- Checking with a camera
- Electrical appliances like hair straighteners
- Driving route and checking the car
- Re-reading text

- Pregnancy
- Illness and conditions
- HIV and AIDS
- Schizophrenia
- Sexual arousal
- Valuable items like a wallet, phone, and purse.

Checking is most times carried out multiple times, sometimes hundreds of times, and this might last for an hour or even longer, causing a major effect on the person's life, work, social occasion, school, and other appointments. This can have a strong influence on a person's attitude to hold relationships and jobs, which is a reason why the phrase says 'a little bit OCD' is offensive and not accurate. Another importance of checking compulsion is that they can sometimes harm objects that are persistently being prodded, pulled, or even over tightened.

Contamination

Phobia of being dirty and contamination is worries that are obsessional, at times, fear is the contamination may cause harm to a loved one or yourself. The common compulsion might be to clean, avoid or wash, other contamination obsession worries and compulsion include:

- Eating in public locations
- Crowds
- Money
- Public toilets
- Shaking hands
- Public telephones
- GP Surgery/ Hospital
- Chemicals
- Staircase banister
- Bathroom
- Teeth brushing
- Places

• Outside air

The washing or cleaning is at times, carried out multiple times, often followed by rituals of repeating washing the body until the person knows that it is clean, instead of someone without OCD will clean or wash only once until they observe that they are clean. This can have a serious influence on the person's ability to keep relationships and jobs, and there is also a physical health impact of consistently scrubbing and cleaning on the skin, most importantly the hands. Someone might scrub until their hands bleed. While others have gone as far as bathing in bleach.

A person might also try as much as possible to keep away from places, objects, or even people if they experience fears from contaminations. There are also implications of cost due to the persistent purchase and use of cleaning products, and also of items, particularly electrical items like mobile phones that are damaged through too much liquid damage.

Mental Contamination

Additionally, there are more familiar types of OCD contaminations that involve someone washing their hands repetitively after coming in contact with potential dirty environments or objects; there is also a less known form which is called 'mental contamination.' Researchers have just started to get a basic understanding of mental contamination. The feelings of mental contamination share some important qualities with contact contamination, both having distinctive features. Feelings of mental contamination can be brought about most times when a person felt that they were treated badly, mentally, physically, via verbally or critically abusive remarks. It is sometimes as if they are meant to feel or act dirty and this creates a feeling of internal uncleanliness or even its absence of any physical contact with a harmful/dirty object. A characteristic of mental contamination is that the source is almost like that of normal human contamination which is caused by physical contact, but its own is caused by contact with inanimate objects. This might result in engaging in compulsive and repetitive attempts to clean the dirt away by washing and showering which lays the resemblance with traditional contamination OCD return; the major difference is that contaminated feeling will not need to come from physical contact, at times, there is a lonely feeling with mental contamination.

Ruminations

Ruminations is a terminology that is used to describe all obsessional intrusive thoughts, and defining rumination likely assist in encouraging the belief that "a deep or known thought about anything," but this is misleading from an OCD view. Using the context of OCD, rumination is trained to extend thinking about a theme, question that is not productive or not directed. Unlike obsessional thoughts, ruminations are just not objectionable and do not yield instead of resisting, so many ruminations are based on philosophical, metaphysical topics, religious such as life after death, the nature of morality, the origins of the universe and many more.

An example of this is when a person dwells on a time-consuming question: 'is everyone looking good?' They will also think about this for a very long period, going over it in their minds with different arguments, consideration, and contemplating compelling evidence. Another example is just someone that thinks about what will happen once they are dead, they will weigh up different possibilities theoretically, visualizing how heaven or hell might look, or other worlds, and they'll try to think about what other philosophers and scientist has discussed about death. With ruminations, it predictably never leads to a solution or satisfactory conclusion, and someone seems to be deeply rooted, thoughtful and also detached.

Preparing the Way for Your Patient

Before directing a patient for CBT, questions about the practitioner's level of training should be asked (Ph.D. or PsyD are better). Also, theoretical methods (Cognitive Behavioral vs. others, like Humanistic or Psychodynamic), and experience working with patients that have OCD should be asked. One of the questions that should be asked when meeting a clinician is "Will you allow your patients to be vulnerable to situations that bring about rituals while you are trying to refrain him or her from engaging in them?"

What Your Patients Can Expect?

CBT is a form of psychological treatment specifically based on acquiring knowledge and cognitive rules. Normally, there will be 12-16 sessions; though every individual function goes a long way in determining how long the treatment will go. The treatment can be stopped when you noticed that there is a great deal of change in the symptoms for at least four continuous weeks. Later on, timely booster sessions are useful in maintaining the benefits and prevent fallbacks.

Chapter 11: CBT for Intrusive Thoughts and OCD

Using the context of OCD, where one suffers so much from thoughts that are obsessional that is repetitive, disturbing, horrific and offensive. For example, the thought that constantly comes to you about hurting someone you love in a violent way, and this does not involve a specific compulsion, they are called intrusive thoughts, and they are often called "Pure O."

Everyone who is alive has had intrusive thoughts and of course it has been proved that everyone who has OCD will have "intrusive thoughts" which can either be positive or negative. Thinking about winning the lottery is also an intrusive thought, but it is just a great one. From the view of the OCD, it is always assumed that the thoughts are not repeating (constant) and pleasant, and it is also accepted that when you are talking about OCD 'intrusive thoughts' is of the type that will be listed below which will cover topics, but more specialization common to OCD covers the following:

Relationship Intrusive Thoughts

Relationship intrusive thoughts have preoccupied doubts that arise over how standard a relationship is; personal security of one's partner is one of the major focus for thoughts that are obsessional.

Obsessional thoughts include:

- Constantly needing to seek reassurance and the approval of one's partner.

- Doubts that a partner is faithful.

• Questioning one's sexuality, and having feelings, impulses, and thoughts about being attracted to members of the same sex.

• Constantly examining partners depth of feelings, putting the partner and the relationship under watch and always finding faults.

• The constant questioning, constant analysis of the relationship or partners often places a deep strain on the relationship and outcome when the person has OCD is that the person might break the relationship to stop anxiety and doubts which is often repeating itself with other types of relationship.

• Doubts of infidelity from another partner.

Sexual Sensitive Thoughts

Sexual sensitive thoughts are thoughts that are obsessive about causing harm that is not done purposefully. This could be thoughts of inappropriately harming children sexually. It's not intentional, or it could be a consistent thought about someone in a sexual way.

The major focus of obsessional sexual thoughts includes: is the consistent questioning of how someone can be and this are the major focus for obsessional thoughts. They include;

• The thoughts of touching a child inappropriately.

• The consistent analysis and the questioning of your sexual capability, or the thoughts about being attracted to children, are the most likely two disturbing mental parts of OCD, and because of the nature of the thoughts, many people that are suffering this are not willing to seek for assistance of any health professional and fears of being labeled.

- Fear of being attracted to people that are of the same sex (homosexuals) or fear of those who are gay, they have a fear of being attracted to people of opposite sex.

- Intrusive sexual thoughts about God, religious figures, or even about saints.

- Fear of being a pedophile and then attracted sexually to them.

Someone who experiences these types of intrusive thoughts will avoid public places like the shopping mall to keep away from getting close to children. They will also have to stay away from their siblings. For parents that experience this type of illness, they will try as much as possible to stay away from hugging or bathing their kids, which will result in emotional discomfort for both the children and the parents.

Magical Thinking about Intrusive Thoughts

Magical thinking about intrusive thoughts is having fears about thinking something negative will make it more likely for it to occur which is often referred to as 'thoughts action fusion.' The people surrounded by intrusive bad thoughts are the ones suffering, they try to take them away by going through rituals that are magical. They are conventionally strange in style and time-consuming, and they may also be involved in events or action links that may not be related to each other. Example, having the thoughts like 'I might strangle someone' is also seen as someone who is guilty of actually committing the crime. Another example is that you have terrible thoughts about your car having a ghastly accident, it might also increase the chance of it, or someone has a feeling that if they do not count 1-10 'just right' something bad might happen to a family member.

Other examples that are given below are;

- A loved one's death can be predicted.

- One can cause much harm to someone with their thoughts or carelessness.

- Attending one's funeral can bring death.

- Whatever comes to your mind can be true.

- Breaking a chain letter can bring about bad luck.

- Stepping on cracks in the pavement can allow bad things to occur.

- Hearing the word 'death' will mean the opposite like repeating the word 'life' to resist death.

- Certain days also have good or bad luck with them.

- Certain number or color has either good or bad luck that is associated with it.

In the examples above, the thoughts and events could be linked but one who has OCD will believe that the possibility of this occurring does not exist and this will lead to deep stress and anxiety. As a result of this, their internal compulsive behaviors can often keep them from interacting with other people at this time.

Religious Intrusive Thoughts

Religious intrusive thoughts with OCD are often fixed on areas of great importance, religion and matters that concern religious practice are the basic candidates for OCD obsessions. Often it is known as scrupulosity, examples of intrusive religious thoughts are listed below;

- That person has lost touch with God or their beliefs in some ways.

- Prayers are recited and omitted wrongly.

- One is doing something sinful.

- Certain prayers can be said repetitively.

- That the person has flouted religious laws that concern dress, speech, and moderations.

- Intrusive sexual thoughts about religious figures, saints, and God.

- Repeated blasphemous thoughts.

- Sins that are committed will never be forgiven by God, and one will end up in hell.

- One can have bad thoughts in a religious building.

- One will yell blasphemous words aloud in a religious location.

Intrusive bad thoughts occur during the time that prayers will be spoiled, corrupt or cancel the value of the activities, the consistent questioning, and analysis of one's faith will place a great strain on their beliefs, and this will prevent someone who derives peace from his or her religion. This will make some people avoid the church and all religious thoughts for fear of their thoughts.

Violent Intrusive Thoughts

Intrusive violent thoughts have obsessive fears of carrying out lots of violence against people you truly love or every other person. These thoughts include;

- Jumping in front of a moving car

- Thoughts about accidentally touching someone badly with the aim of touching them.

- Harming children or loved ones.

- Acting on unwanted impulse; for example, stabbing someone or running someone over.

- Poisoning the food of a loved one (compulsion will mean not cooking for the family).

- Killing innocent people

- Utilizing sharp objects such as kitchen knives.

Those suffering from this type of fear most of the time allow themselves to feel like a bad person for just having bad thoughts, they believe that having these thoughts means that they truly have the capacity of carrying it out.

The consistent questioning and analysis of this disturbing part of the OCD become more upsetting, and because of the nature of his or her thoughts, those undergoing this are reluctant to open up even to their health professional for help having a fear of being exposed. A person who has this form of intrusive thoughts will avoid places like the shopping centers and other vital areas where social interaction is required to prevent having close contacts with people that will initiate obsessional thoughts.

Body-focused Obsession (sensorimotor OCD)

Hyperawareness of the sensation of a specific body is also known to as sensorimotor obsessions. Symptoms include;

- Eye floaters/visual distractors, obsessive fixation on eye floaters

- Swallowing/salivation, focusing on how well to swallow the amount of salivation produced or sensation of swallowing itself.

- Awareness of a specific body part, example, the perception of the side of one's nose when trying to read.

- Breathing, obsessions whether you are breathing is shallow or deep, or the focus is on some other sensation of breathing.

- Blinking, obsessive fixation on blinking.

This form of OCD should not be muddled up with BDD whereby the obsession is much more about the defects that are noticed within the part of the body. The intrusive thoughts are repetitive, and they are not developed voluntarily, they make the person who suffers uncomfortable from excessive discomfort which is the reason why they are having the thoughts in the first place, and the feelings of having the thoughts in the first place can be terrifying.

However, what we know is that people are more interested in the obsessive-compulsive disorder and they might act on these thoughts, partly because they are offensive, and they can go very far from preventing it from happening.

To those suffering and those who are not suffering from it, the thoughts and the fears associated with OCD tends to be shocking and meaningful at times. Nevertheless, the fact that they are thoughts does not mean that they are developed voluntarily. Neither fantasies or impulses should be acted upon. The various information could be a physical or mental compulsion, and it does not remain helpful.

Symmetry and Orderliness

There is a need for everything that is put together in symmetric order, and 'just' right is the compulsion, the fears that are obsessive might just want you to know that everything you feel is 'just' right to stop discomfort or often prevent harm from happening. Examples include;

• Having everything spotless with no smudges on windows, on marks and surfaces less about contaminating and cleaning extra well for neatness and being right.

• Clothes.

• Arranging things neatly and at all times.

• Having your books and CD's lined up perfectly in a row on a bookshelf.

• Tinned cans.

• Having pictures well arranged.

• Having your clothes hung on rails and all facing the same way.

• Neatness.

The people that are affected spend more time trying to know the symmetry 'just right,' and this makes it more time consuming and this results in being very late to appointments and work. They can be draining both physically and mentally. If the compulsion is going to take more time, the person suffering might not want to prevent contacts at home to stop the symmetry, being interrupted and can result in having lesser impacts on social interactions and relationships.

The list shows the known common type of OCD and the fears that accompany it, but this is not a drawn list, and there will be other types of OCD. If the impacts are functioning properly, it can represent the principal part in the diagnosis of an obsessive-compulsion disorder; then it is vital for you to consult a doctor and get a proper diagnosis.

Regardless of the type of OCD one might be suffering from, the 3 following aspects are there generally, and they are; Triggers, Reassurance, and Avoidance.

1. Trigger

This is the basic source of obsessional worry which can either be a place, person, or objects that allows for obsession, a compulsive feeling, or the feelings of distress. A trigger might be internal thoughts or physical objects; for example, someone who has the obsessed feeling about stabbing someone whenever he or she comes in contact with sharp objects, seeing that the knife will always provoke the compulsions and obsessions.

Also, to avoid several hours of pain, the person will always keep away from knives, an example of an internal mental trigger is when one experiences distress obsessions about death every time the thoughts about his late father comes, the memory of their late father acts as a trigger for obsessional thoughts. What happens is that people with OCD discovered their compulsion and obsessions physically and mentally draining, scary, and frightening. They have to go to great lengths to avoiding the triggers during the time of compulsions and obsessions.

1. Avoidance

This is an occasional compulsive, and it happens where the individual with OCD keeps away from objects, places, or a person that can trigger OCD. This will be a way of preventing the anguish, distress, and the time used in undergoing the rituals. Examples include those who checks compulsion that might not be able to stay away from situations or task that will elevate the rate at which they are responsible and are not safe.

• Someone with obsessional thoughts can have the feeling of stabbing their children and will always avoid the use of scissors, knives, or any sharp objects.

• Someone who has a fear of having HIV or AIDS avoid going to places like London in which in their minds is associated with HIV or AIDS.

1. Reassurance

The person having issues with OCD will often times need reassurance that the feelings around them are not real, this reassurance can come from someone they love or through sources like the Google or news outlets. Especially if the worry is getting to the point of crimes or accidents. Frequently, the obsessional worry might be to someone you love, and you think something bad might happen to them, they will repeatedly check on their loved ones to see if they are doing fine. Another obsessional fear results in reassurance seeking for compulsive worries that their partners might not have the feeling for them or they will do something terrible to their loved one.

Various terms and acronyms can be used with the OCD family which can lead to confusions.

Acronyms commonly used for OCD

Ritual

One of the terms causing confusion is the word 'ritual' in which other people including the health professionals get confused with and then describe it as 'compulsion.' While this is certain about ritual being a compulsive behavior (mental or physical), it is just a specific compulsive behavior that is more than a set pattern of behaviors will certainly define the start and finish point. Example, massage the left side of your face, your forehead and the right side, in many cases, when the person undergoing rituals stops during the time of the ritual steps, then their OCD decides when to start their ritual over again.

Spike

Spike is also a terminology that confuses mainly those with OCD who try to get more information about it online research about it online; there tends to be two major use of this term. With people who have OCD on OCD board online; there tends to be two major use of this terms. The first one is when it is used in explaining the starting obsession 'trigger' that leads to anxiety and discomfort, example, an individual that is scared of hitting a cyclist while driving will use the term 'spike' to explain the cyclist that is moving ahead of them, and that triggers the compulsion and obsession. Another use of this term is in the OCD format is used when explaining the increase in the anxiety levels, and it is caused by obsessional thoughts. Using the example given of person that is afraid of hitting a cyclist while driving will tend to understand that the cyclist is the reason for the obsessive thoughts rising 'spike' activities.

Presently, there is no particular way to describe what spike is officially all about, but what spike means generally is that it is used to describe the joining together of OCD obsessions, triggers, or discomforts caused by anxiety which is the reasons to remove the confusions. We try as much as possible to stop using the word 'spike' in writing if there is no loss of meanings or context. So many people use terminologies to refer to different types of OCD, it is noteworthy that there is no official definition in medical science, and it is usually used by the OCD community in OCD meetings using the internet. One of the main issues with these terminologies is that they are mostly confusing since they mean something different to entirely different people. More information on the 3 major purposes on the main acronyms are;

POCD (Pedophile OCD)

This describes the postpartum and the parental OCD and 'Pure O.' Nevertheless, this is accepted widely to pedophile OCD, in few cases, we are aware of the users that use OCD consciously as a means of avoiding saying pedophile. Getting used to this line of thought is the first step in accepting that it exists. which is trying to get used to the thoughts is the first step of accepting it.

ROCD (Relationship OCD)

It is commonly used in describing the ruminating and religious OCD, which is used widely to accept mean relationship OCD because there are no medical meanings attached to it and prevent people from being confused. So, we try to stay away from acronyms whenever you are writing and make sure that you ensure that there is no loss of meaning or context. Usually, we discourage most people from trying it and on a different occasion, the use results in the delay of assessing their treatments. This mostly happens when a patient looks for a specialist in (H/P/R) OCD, but they are unable to find any since they are not recognized in medical science. There are no recommendations given yet to any specialist to specialize in any of the types of OCD since all OCD have the same way of treating the addressed C and O part.

This might not prevent progress in tackling and getting rid of OCD because it is certain that OCD that changes periodically and changes like a chameleon (note that it only focuses on objects or individuals that are special to us), as with the changes, so does the OCD. So, it is very important to treat OCD and not (H/P/R). One major point to note is that they will be treated using Cognitive Behavioral Therapy.

HOCD (Homosexual OCD)

This is not one of the helpful terminologies because it is meant for the people who are scared of being homosexual, we know that it is the same OCD that affects the homosexual with obsessional fears while they are not actually homosexual. A preferable acronym to be used is SOCD (Sexual orientation OCD)

If you are experiencing attacks frequently and you have been diagnosed with another type of anxiety disorder, it is possible to develop unintentional non-adaptive terrible methods of coping with the situation.

Treatment of OCD Intrusive Thoughts Using CBT

Those who have intrusive thoughts gotten from OCD complex PTSD intrusive thought gain from mind exercise but this usually needs treatment and self-help too. CBT has proved effective in patients (70%) with OCD. Through CBT, patients have a way of dealing with their fears and eliminate compulsions; it is an essential treatment of detoxifying the mind wholly. Modified CBT methods for treating intrusive thoughts and OCD include;

- Situational exposure
- Taking a self-report questionnaire like the OCD intrusive thoughts tests
- Gathering evidence to challenge the deep beliefs patients has

- Role play stimulation with electronic cueing
- Intentional thought exposure
- Refocus the brain through mental education
- Deciding on the thought process each person undergoes
- Non-judgmental acceptance

Chapter 12: CBT for Mental Health and Exercise

Cognitive Tools & Exercise

Various CBT tools focus on the changing and challenging patient's dysfunctional method of thinking since CBT therapists are also taught to make use of a top-down method, first of all, working with the patient's thought, activities, and cognitive exercise are of useful importance. To change the downward spiral or reverse mental health disorder, patients will know about the cognitive restructuring and begin to use tools like the dysfunctional thought records and the ABCD strategies.

Behavioral Tools & Exercise

Besides the cognitive tools and exercise, CBT therapist teaches their client's various behavioral methods that might help change the problematic thoughts and limiting beliefs into life-affirming alternatives. By taking a strong action that is against what they may tell themselves, individuals are more able to compile the evidence that goes against harming cognitive patterns. Very good examples of behavioral tools are behavioral experiments, behavioral rehearsal, and behavioral activation.

Tools from Third-Wave Therapies

There are additional ways of various means of innovative third wave therapeutic methods that are gotten from CBT, and this provides new additions to the CBT toolbox. While not all the therapist use what is known to be considered to be a third-wave activities or exercise, it is of note to them because it can help achieve dreams, specific tools that are found in the third-wave therapies like the Acceptance and Commitment Therapy (ACT) and Mindfulness-Based Cognitive therapy (MBCT) is very useful for our endeavors.

Mental Health Ailments that may improve with CBT

Handle grief

The client and therapist additionally consider how thoughts and behaviors affect emotions. For instance, if someone thinks that nothing could work out to them in life, they can withdraw from others and also prevent brand new chances. This, subsequently, can lead to feelings of increased despair, emptiness, and stress. This is sometimes known as a "vicious circle" of emotions, thoughts, and behaviors.

Try to be patient: Even though CBT performs fast for lots of individuals, it's an ongoing procedure that's essentially life-long. There are always approaches to boost, feel happier, and also treat others and yourself better, so exercise being individual. Remind yourself there is no finish line. Give your self-credit for placing effort into confronting your issues immediately, and attempt and look at "slip ups" as certain parts of the process and mastering procedure.

PTSD

CBT is most commonly applied to mood disorders (for example, depression) and anxiety disorders. It is likewise used to aid individuals who have chemical use complications, personality disorders, eating disorders, sexual issues, and psychosis. It is properly delivered into the personal, couples, and group formats.

A psychotherapist can be an overall period, instead of a job title or hint of education, instruction or licensure. Examples of psychotherapists consist of psychiatrists, psychologists, certified professional counselors, licensed social workers, certified marriage and family therapists, psychiatric nurses, or even other certified practitioners with mental wellness coaching.

Your therapist may persuade you to discuss your thinking and emotions and what's troubling you. Do not be concerned if you simply still discover that it's tough to open about your feelings. Your therapist will assist you to gain greater confidence and comfort.

The Downward Spiral of Mental Disorder

A mother and daughter crying with their heads bowed down, it looks like a tragic event took place in their lives leading to a downward spiral towards negative mental health disorder. The CBT therapist can give their patients good treatment methods on an individual basis. This, however, does not mean that mental illness brings themselves in separate ways; there is much disorder that is being influenced by genes or life experiences that develops closely in a systematic approach.

For those who are suffering from depression or anxiety; an example, bad events or set of successful order typically set of successful events typically leads to the beginning of cognitive behavioral and emotional symptoms, especially when an individual cannot stop or reverse their anxiousness or depressive response they will start spiraling downwards towards a full mental disorder.

The CBT examined previously to assist in showing the downward spiral mental health disorders because it shows us how the problematic thoughts, emotional response, behaviors, and emotional response can respectively influence another by needing medical assistance. The damaged cognitive ways of an individual who loses a premature loved one, example, this can be of negative influence as their behaviors and emotions are ways that lead to a serious depressive disorder.

Certainly, grieving the loss of someone you love can be healthy to some extent but if the individual affected is unable to break the cycle of cognitions, behaviors, and emotions negatively affecting one another, they will be spiral downward to a state of fear. To assist them from a depressive state, a CBT therapist will represent various cognitive behavioral activities that are the opposite direction of the downward spiral.

It should be known that CBT therapist first works with the parent's level behavior and cognition, they will often have to assist them in discovering the change core value, challenge and underlying assumptions of how the world will move them in the direction of stabilized mental health.

Chapter 13: CBT for Self-Monitoring & Progress Evaluation

Two most essential CBT methods are the practices of self-monitoring and examining progress, by raising self-awareness and most times assess the state of one's being, individuals are also able to discover the faulty cognitions, limiting the core values, patterns of dysfunctional thinking, and behavioral hindrances. With this powerful insight, CBT therapist will guide the parents in taking steps that will prevail whether a behavior or mental obstacle.

The practices of self-monitoring and evaluation are the heart of CBT, just as every individual can prevail over mental illness by becoming conscious of the challenging behaviors and improving the probability for success by enhancing and monitoring the actions and thoughts. Great practices that can widely increase the awareness of the inhibiting thoughts, harmful behaviors and limiting beliefs that act as roadblocks on the path of success is the third strategy of mindful meditation.

While undertaking practices of SMART goals, self-monitoring, action plans, and self-evaluation, it is typically enough to make individuals achieve success and decrease the amount of time it takes to achieve goals by using several CBT tools. Basing decisions on and attaching to general psychological governing principles like the mind-body connection and the law of effects and cause, just as the CBT practitioners assist their patients to do, we can confidently transform our lives in the most necessary ways. After we begin to spin the positive spiral of personal growth with the CBT methods, the following will be used to build our starting momentum.

The CBT Toolbox

There are a wide variety of CBT tools that therapist use to improve the mental health of their patients, unlike some treatment methods, cogni-

tive behaviors therapy helps to limit the way parents rely on the medications rather than focusing on establishing a behavioral and cognitive
change through various modes of exercise and activities. After establishing a case formulation gotten from initial therapeutic communications with their patients, a CBT therapist will start recommending several cognitive and behavioral practices that are found within the toolbox of CBT. The exercise from the toolbox is vital due to the long-term
necessity to give patients the resources to act as their therapist later in
the future.

While there are several activities and exercises that may be used
for a specific medical case, or favored by a particular therapist, there
is an accepted range set for CBT methods based on their effectiveness
and popularity. It is with standardized tools and techniques that can be
used to enhance the success of achieving our aim or goals. We will examine, but it will be useful to gain more understanding of how CBT
therapists frame their treatments methods.

Using CBT to Achieve Success

Since the basis of CBT is upon several psychological truths that are applied to everyone, they all can use the CBT methods to improve our
level of wellbeing. Also, a CBT therapist assists their patients to change
their downward spiral mental health; it is possible to use CBT tools as a
springboard to success. One ideological way to meditate on using CBT
for personal growth is to envision a scale that ranges from -5 to 0, represent every individual who has mental illness while the range of 0 to
5 represents healthy minded individuals that pursue high levels of life
satisfaction. It is obvious to note that implementing CBT methods to
improve your self-worth, you will learn fast on how positive emotions
and thoughts can spiral you towards great success.

Defining Success

While there is an endless number of a personal growth goal that you can use CBT methods to achieve, the first step is to know which one will guarantee you success. Unfortunately, many people fall victim to assuming that materials, money, possessions, and social status will give them the satisfaction that is needed only to discover that limited happiness is achieved from them.

SMART Goals & Action Plan

The therapist and clients work together to establish a SMART goal that is (Specific, Measurable, Achievable, Relevant & Time-Bound) and make an achievable plan that assists towards accomplishing their desire. Typically, both the patient and therapist will meet together on a scheduled basis to review, update the client's formulations, goals, and action plan.

We know what success is all about, we can establish the SMART goals. Generally, we may consider having goals in a number of the following steps; Personal & Intellectual, Health Fitness, Spiritual, Financial & Professional Developments and Communication. Also, personal qualities like social intelligence and emotional may be difficult to measure; these are some of the most vital and rewarding goals to help because they are needed to achieve some extraordinary things. Just by committing yourself to also focusing on targets that are intrinsic and desires, in addition to this external success, you will be able to discover the life-satisfaction that is craved for. Before moving to the action plan, you need to consider your objectives using SMART goals. There is no reason to feel discouraged if you have the aim to achieve something monumental, you will have to put the bigger aspirations down into smaller, time-bound and measurable. You will have to reduce the bigger goals into smaller, time-bound and measurable goals.

The next step in using the process of CBT for success, which is to be considered the final step in the initial phase, would be to establish a management plan that might allow you to monitor your progress. While deciding on the methods that will be used to break down specific objectives will be for a particular individual option that is mainly based on situations and plans, the most necessary thing to do is to review and update your appropriate measurable and time-bound action plan.

Chapter 14: How CBT Deals With Things

There are just so many methods of achieving CBT or tools that can be used in CBT. This therapy extends from the background of the therapy to daily life experiences. The nine methods have been listed below, and some are known to be an effective and common practice of CBT.

- Unraveling Cognitive Distortions

This one of the main aim of Cognitive Behavioral Therapy and this can be done without or with the aid of a therapist, just to unfold the hold of the Cognitive aberrations, first be conscious of the aberrations that you are most likely to be exposed to, part of which involves you must be able to identify and challenge our injurious automatic thoughts, which from time to time fall into any categories listed beforehand.

This is one of the main aims of Cognitive Behavioral Therapy and it can be done without or with the aid of a therapist. To unravel cognitive distortions, you must first be conscious of the distortions you may likely be exposed to. It also involves you identifying and challenging those negative thoughts that pop up in our minds from time to time.

- Exposure and Response Prevention

This kind of method is specifically effective for people that undergo hardship of obsessive-compulsive disorder (OCD), you must be able to practice this type of method by being vulnerable to whatever evokes a compulsive behavior, but also do your best to hold back from writing about it and the behavior. It is possible to add together journaling with these methods to get how this method can make you feel.

- Journaling

This method is a means of "collecting data" concerning our thoughts and moods, this journal must contain the period of the mood or thought, it's the source, the range or the degree of strength among so many other things. This necessary CBT tools and methods can assist us in learning our emotional tendencies and thoughts, find out how they are replaced, how they adapt, or the way at which they are able to cope with it.

- Cognitive Restructuring

Immediately, you have been able to know exactly what the aberrations are or the views that are not accurate, you then start to understand how the aberrations started and what exactly made you believe in it. When you know that it is a behavior that is harmful or injurious, you can start to confront it. Example, when you have the consciousness that you have a job that pays well and earns you respect within the society, but then you lost paying job, you will start to feel terrible about yourself. Rather than accepting this belief that makes you think bad about yourself, you can think about the occasion that allows you feel like a well know respectable person, a belief that may not have come to your mind before.

- Nightmare Exposure and Rescripting

Nightmare vulnerability and rescripting are designed specifically to those who are going through difficult moments of a nightmare; this method is also known to be almost the same as interceptive exposure, in that the nightmare has been evoked which then bring up emotions. The therapist and the client must work together to know what type of emotions are desired and how to develop new images to follow the emotions that are desired.

- Progressive Muscle Relaxation

This is a known method to those that practice being mindful, also the same as the body scan; this method will teach you how to relax a type of your muscle group at a period whereby your body falls under the state of necessary CBT methods and relaxation tools. It's possible to use a YouTube video, audio guidance, or just using your mind to know how to practice these methods and this can be most helpful for calming nerves and soothing an unfocused and busy mind.

- Introspective Exposure

This method is designed to treat anxiety and panic; it includes being exposed to bodily excitement that is feared in order to evoke responses activating unhealthy beliefs that are known to be connected with the excitements, preserve the sensations without avoiding them or distraction and this allows acquiring new things about the sensations. It is designed to help the person suffering to understand that the symptoms of this panic are not harmful, though, it can be very uncomfortable.

- Play the script until the End

This method is basically for those that are undergoing anxiety and fears, using this type of method, the individual that is exposed to crippling anxiety or fears controls experimental thoughts where they are able to think about the result of the worst-case models. Allowing this scenario to assist the client to know that even when it seems, there will be fears, it will turn out very good. This method will assist those with anxiety and fears to believe that their worst fears would eventually turn out to be good experience.

- Relaxed Breathing

This is another method which is not known to CBT but is very popular among the mindful practitioners; there are many obvious ways to relax and also bring orderliness and calmness to your breathing, which gives you an edge to see your problems from a balanced position, bringing about more efficient and logical decision-making. These methods can assist those who are going through a range of mental afflictions and illness which includes OCD, depression, panic disorder, anxiety and how they can be practiced without or with the aid of a therapist.

Getting the Most out of it

CBT can be applied daily to principles and methods that surround a wide range of problems. Relaxation skills are very much essential in any stressful circumstance which includes; speaking in public, having an argument with partners, feeling angry at a stubborn teenager, taking a test, sleep problems, and road rage.

Problem-solving methods can be useful in dealing with related issues that concern work that is prioritizing, a demanding boss and time management or interpersonal difficulties or relationship problems. Some people have some attitudes that are irrational, and this creates unnecessary bad feelings in certain situations.

So, anyone can also gain from disputing and identifying unfounded beliefs and this result in experiences that have less bad emotions, and this can be more effective in their lives. Exposure exercise is not just helpful in phobias but as a way of removing all types of fears which include fears of making mistakes, fears of animals, and fear of heights. Additionally, CBT techniques are more useful to every one of our lives whether they have a psychological disorder or those who deal with real-life solutions.

Chapter 15: Final Thoughts on Cognitive Behavioral Therapy

CBT was initially created to assist people afflicted by depression; however today it is utilized to boost and control different types of emotional illnesses and symptoms, for example, anxiety, bipolar illness, post-traumatic stress illness, obsessive-compulsive disease, addictions, and eating disorders.

CBT techniques will also be favorable to just about everybody, for example, people with no type of emotional disease but with chronic anxiety, inferior moods, and habits they want to do their job with.

Scientific tests have discovered that in most those who have accomplished CBT and then undergone brain scans proves that CBT is capable of favorably adjusting physical structures inside mental performance.

CBT can get the job done fast, assisting people to feel better and experience lessened symptoms within a quick period (a few months, for instance).

When many kinds of therapy could take some months or even years to become beneficial, the average quantity of CBT periods clients receive is 16.

CBT often requires the individual finishing "homework" duties independently amongst therapy sessions, which is one reason benefits come so fast.

In addition to prep being done from the people while they truly are alone, cognitive behavioral therapists also utilize instructions, such as coughing and "vulnerability therapy" throughout periods.

CBT is extremely interactive and collaborative. The therapist's role would always be there to listen, teach and encourage, while the individual's role is to be more open and expressive.

What Next For the Future of CBT?

Several strategies and benefit of CBT have been discussed so far in this book. Here is a recap and some closing thoughts about CBT and reasons why it may be best for you.

The evolution of cultural adaptations into CBT is still at the beginning phases. CBT hinges predominantly on the values supported from the dominant civilization. Back in North America, these values incorporate assertiveness, personal independence, verbal power, logic and behavior change. But specific manuals are created for adapting CBT to Chinese-Americans and Haitian-American adolescents.

Cognitive behavioral therapy (CBT) can be just a usual sort of conversation therapy (psychotherapy). You work with a mental wellness counselor (psychotherapist or therapist) in a structured manner, attending quite a limited amount of sessions. CBT makes it possible to become aware of wrong or unwanted thoughts, and that means you can view challenging scenarios more certainly and respond in your mind in a better way.

In CBT, the therapist and the customer come together to determine unhelpful patterns of thinking and behavior. By way of instance, somebody might just notice the bad things that happen to these and never notice the positive things. Or, someone could put unrealistic specifications on their own, such as "creating blunders in the office is improper." Also, it is essential to determine curable behaviors that take outward symptoms, such as avoiding particular situations and withdrawing from others.

It is crucial that you decide to try and view predicaments as rationally, clearly and realistically as you possibly can. It is helpful to think about different people's perspectives, question your premises, and see whether there is something crucial you may be missing or dismissing.

How Many CBT Sessions Will You Need to Get the Desired Result?

CBT is commonly regarded as short-term therapy—approximately 10 to 20 sessions. You along with your therapist can talk about how many sessions may be appropriate for you personally.

At your first session, your therapist will collect information on you personally and get exactly what concerns you may have. The therapist will likely inquire regarding your present and past physical and emotional health to gain a deeper comprehension of your circumstance. Your therapist can discuss if you might benefit from additional treatment as well, like medication.

The therapist works together with clients to tackle unfavorable perspectives the consumer retains about itself, the world and the future, which may bring about feelings of despair.

Is CBT limited in Any Way?

CBT doesn't have limitations because it can be adapted to solve various issues. Carefully assembled exercises are used to support and modify feelings and behaviors. Some therapies focus more on notions, and also some aspects focus a lot more on behaviors. When someone has trouble identifying and challenging mental issues, the therapist might focus on addressing behaviors like avoidance, withdrawal, or poor interpersonal knowledge.

On the other hand, if this sort of behaviors is less noticeable, the therapist may focus on low-self-esteem.

The very first session is also an opportunity for you to interview your therapist to find out whether he or she's going to be a good fit for you personally.

Learning About Your Emotional Health Condition

Recognize troubling situations or illnesses in your life is part of therapy. These may include problems such as a medical condition, divorce, despair, anger or symptoms of mental illness. You and your therapist may dedicate some time to identify the problems and aims that you want to focus on. Cognitive behavioral therapy may be achieved one-on-one, or even in categories together with family members with those that have similar difficulties.

What You May Anticipate

CBT typically specializes in special issues, utilizing a goal-oriented strategy. Since you proceed through the therapy approach, your therapist might ask you to do "assignments"—tasks, examining through or practices that build on what you find out during your regular therapy sessions—and invite you to utilize exactly what you are learning into your normal lifestyle.

Identify Strategies to Manage Emotions

Cognitive behavioral therapy can be utilized to take care of a vast variety of issues. It is usually the preferred kind of psychotherapy as it could quickly help you determine and cope with challenges that are specific. It usually requires fewer periods than different forms of therapy and can be done in a coordinated way.

Ways to Practice Cognitive Behavioral Therapy Techniques on Your Own

1. Describe your present obstacles

The very first thing to do is to identify what's causing you to worry, un-happiness and unease. Maybe you're feeling resentful toward someone, fearful of failure, or stressed about being refused socially in some way. You might realize that you have persistent stress, indicators of melan-choly, or are fighting to forgive somebody for a past event. When you can recognize this and become aware of your main barrier, then you have the power to start work on overcoming it.

1. Be wary of your emotions, thoughts, and beliefs about these issues.

When you have determined the issues to focus on, your therapist will encourage you to discuss your thinking regarding these. This could consist of celebrating what you know about experience, your perspec-tive of a situation, and your self-beliefs, other people and events. Your therapist will recommend you keep a journal of your thoughts.

1. Be able to look after yourself securely

Reshape incorrect or negative thinking. Your therapist will likely encourage you to inquire if an opinion of a situation is situated in fact or in an erroneous perception of what's going on. This step might be difficult. You may have long-standing ways of thinking in your own life as well as yourself. Together with exercise, very beneficial thinking, and behavior styles will grow to be a custom and will not take as much work.

1. Evaluate your queries

Previous to your very first consultation, consider what issues you want to work on while you can also sort out this along with your ther-apist, even having a few senses beforehand can give a starting point.

1. Cope with a medical issue

Even though CBT has been used with kids as young as seven to nine years older, it is most effective with kids with the age of fourteen years. At this age, kids have significantly more improved cognitive skills. Younger kids, or teens and adults, who have cognitive disabilities, generally reply to behavioral plans and ridding of the environment as opposed to a focus on believing.

Make Sure That You know:

- The severity of your outward symptoms
- Identifying scenarios which are frequently averted and steadily approaching dreaded situations
- Popular CBT interventions
- Sexual ailments
- The length of every session

Generally, there is a minimal threat in receiving cognitive behavioral therapy. Because it might research debilitating feelings, emotions, and adventures, you can feel mentally uncomfortable at times. You will shout, be angry or truly feel upset during a session that is tough, or you could even feel drained. You may also threaten to instantly or soon (imminently) hurt yourself or take your own life.

The therapist and client work with each other to anticipate problems and develop successful working strategies. Differentiating and challenging negative thoughts (e.g., "Things never work outside for me personally").

Do your assignments among sessions. If a therapist asks you to browse, maintain a diary, or perform alternative activities outside of your routine therapy sessions to check along with. Doing these homework assignments will allow you to apply what you have learned from the therapy periods.

Stick to your treatment program. In the event you truly feel down or lack motivation, it can be tempting to skip therapy sessions. Doing so can interrupt your progress. Enroll in all sessions and offer a notion about exactly which you want to focus on.

Identifying and engaging in enjoyable activities including hobbies, social pursuits, and physical exercise.

You can apply cognitive behavioral therapy by pinpointing your current challenges, stressful thought recording, forming patterns, and understanding your triggers, discovering how matters are constantly shifting, placing yourself in others' shoes, and thanking yourself for being patient.

One of the primary advantages of patients is that CBT can be continued even after formal sessions with a therapist are over.

Generally, there are few risks in getting CBT. However, you may experience uncomfortable situations at times as it can explore emotions, bad feelings and experiences which may cause you to cry or feel upset during the CBT session. All these are steps and processes to overcome your challenge and develop better coping skills.

Finally, after proper therapy ends, the person could carry on working on researching CBT concepts, applying techniques they've figured out, reading and journaling to aid in lengthening gains and taking care of signs or symptoms.

Conclusion

CBT is a practical therapy to deal with emotional challenges. Various kinds of CBT, like exposure therapy, might ask that you confront predicaments you would rather avert—such as flying in airplanes when you harbor a fear of traveling. This also can result in temporary pressure or anxiety. The impact of CBT therapy in solving most of the disorders and mental issues mentioned in this book cannot be overemphasized as it has been proven to be more effective than other similar therapies.

CBT techniques may also be beneficial for just about everybody, for example, people without a kind of mental disease but who have chronic pressure, poor moods and habits they'd like to work with.

Be honest and open as success with this therapy is dependent on your willingness to share your thoughts, emotions, and experiences, and on being open to fresh insights and means of doing matters. If you're reluctant to discuss certain issues due to debilitating emotions, embarrassment or fears regarding your therapist's response, then allow your therapist to understand regarding your bookings.

CBT isn't the best way for all clients. Those who have significantly more chronic or recurring illness may need repeated interventions. Or they could need a change to tactics apart from CBT to tackle early life adventures along with personal, interpersonal, and identity troubles. And given that CBT can be quite a valuable device in treating emotional health disorders, including depression, post-traumatic stress disorder (PTSD) or an eating disorder. However, perhaps not everybody who benefits from CBT comes with a mental health state. It can be effective tools to assist anyone who learns how to manage difficult daily living conditions.

Before seeing a psychotherapist, check his or her approaches for handling and preventing risky scenarios. You may decide in your mind that you wish to try cognitive behavioral therapy. Or just a health care provider or somebody else may indicate therapy to you. Do not expect instant outcomes. Working on emotional issues can be debilitating and usually requires hard work. It's not unusual to feel worse throughout the initial portion of therapy as you start to confront past and current battles. You may require several sessions before you begin to observe advancement.

This book has touched on every essential aspect of CBT and how to improve your lives and those around you who may be suffering from any emotional challenge. List of cognitive behavioral therapy methods is far from being exhaustible, but this will give you other good ideas on the different methods that are used during cognitive behavioral therapy when working with a therapist and you have been doing your reading about CBT, then you can tell your therapist what type of methods excite you.

I hope you will find strength as you begin to use these therapies to your advantage. I hope it works perfectly for you or other people you recommend it to. I would love to hear your success story after using the steps highlighted in this book.